HOW TO EXPERIENCE REAL HEALTH

Everyday Living

GABRIEL WILSON

0

Copyright © 2023 by Gabriel Wilson

1

TABLE OF CONTENT

Introduction

Emma was a tired lady who desired real health in a busy city. She learned that conscious decision-making is the foundation of true well-being. She enjoyed a hearty meal every morning while soaking in the sun's warm embrace. She chose to take her time walking to work, appreciating the cool wind and taking in the beauty of the outdoors. Emma was grateful, cherished her relationships, and treasured her time spent with her loved ones. She gave her body healthy meals to eat and took part in enjoyable activities that fired her interest. Emma found that genuine health was not a destination but an ongoing journey of conscious living, as a result of placing a high priority on sound sleep and achieving balance. This realization greatly improved Emma's quality of life.

Welcome to Real Health

You have arrived in the actual health world, where normal daily activities take precedence. It's easy to underestimate the impact of our everyday decisions and how they influence our health in an era where fast gratification and quick solutions dominate our focus. This book acts as a beacon, showing the way to achieving true health and serving as a reminder of the influence our daily activities have on our general health.

Why Everyday Living Matters

The importance of daily life: why? Since it serves as the cornerstone of our health, it is important. Our physical, mental, and emotional well-being is impacted by a variety of routines, habits, and lifestyle decisions. Every choice we make affects our well-being, whether it is related to what we eat, what we do, how well we sleep, or how we handle stress.

Understanding the value of daily activities helps us appreciate how much impact we have on our health. It gives us the capacity to make decisions that are in line with our objectives, principles, and aspirations. Real health is about discovering what works best for us as individuals and developing a sustainable lifestyle that fosters energy and balance, rather than about applying to a rigid plan or seeing each other's societal norms. On your life-changing journey, this book wants to be your dependable travel partner. It is intended to give you insightful information, knowledge that is supported by research, and useful tactics that you can use in your everyday life. You will discover a wealth of knowledge to help you on your road to true health, whether you're

looking for advice on diet,
exercise, stress management,
sleep optimization, or
mindfulness.

How This Book Can Help You

This book goes beyond just theoretical ideas. It provides instances and real-life tales of people who have successfully adopted genuine health tenets and gone through astonishing changes. Your inspiration will come from their stories, which demonstrate that anybody who is ready to put themselves first may achieve true health.

11

By the time you finish reading this book, you will have the information, resources, and inspiration needed to start on your unique path to true health. Remember, discovering what satisfies your mind, body, and spirit is more important than obtaining perfection or any other arbitrary goal.

Are you prepared to start this journey, then? Are you prepared to put your daily activities first and achieve true health? If the answer is "yes," then let's explore the transformative potential of adopting a comprehensive strategy for wellness.

Chapter 1: Defining Real Health

The term "real health" refers to a complete and dynamic state of well-being that goes well beyond the simple absence of disease. People may live satisfying lives and realize their full potential thanks to this harmonic balance of the social and physical spheres. Real health embraces energy, resilience, and a strong sense of purpose,

going beyond the narrow idea of a body free of symptoms.
Real health is built on a foundation of physical health. It includes the body's systems operating at their peak potential, including the immunological, digestive, respiratory, cardiovascular, and musculoskeletal systems. Regular exercise, a balanced diet, getting enough sleep, and adopting healthy behaviors like

quitting smoking and drinking too much alcohol all contribute to good physical health. Maintaining a healthy weight, controlling stress, and seeking out preventative treatment to identify and address any health concerns are all part of it.

Additionally, social health is an essential part of actual health, stressing the value of interpersonal relationships and community involvement. Since humans are social creatures, having strong social networks, fulfilling relationships, and a sense of community all contribute to overall well-being. Effective communication, empathy, and a desire to make a constructive contribution to society are all aspects of social health. It acknowledges the need for social assistance during difficult times and the advantages of helping others in return.

Real health recognizes how these dimensions physical and social are interrelated and how they affect one another. It highlights that real health cannot be divided into separate parts but instead results from a seamless fusion of different elements. For instance, exercise releases endorphins, which boost mood and lower stress while also strengthening the body. Similar to how a solid support network may boost

18

emotional toughness, which benefits physical health.

Real health demands a proactive strategy that explains preventative care and lifestyle decisions that put health first. It includes developing self-awareness, establishing practical objectives, and selecting appropriate diet, exercise, and self-care practices. Real Health understands the value of consulting professionals as necessary, including healthcare doctors and other specialists who may assist people on their path to optimum wellness. People may live robust, satisfying lives, reach their full potential, and have a positive effect on the world around them by embracing true health.

The Connection between Mind and Body

Activating Your Inner Power

Philosophers, scientists, and ordinary people have all been interested in the profound and alluring phenomena of the link between mind and body throughout history. The enormous strength and complexity of the human experience are demonstrated by this complicated relationship.

The understanding that the mind and body are not two distinct things but rather components of a single, interconnected whole is at the core of this link. The body's feelings, movements, and physiological processes affect the mind, which in turn is impacted by the body's ideas, beliefs, and emotions. They are entwined in a masterfully planned symphony that affects our perception, actions, and general well-being.

Our thoughts and beliefs have a tremendous amount of power. They can elicit a wide range of feelings, from love and joy to fear and worry, and these emotional states can materialize physically. Consider a period when you were anxious or agitated; recall the fluttering in your stomach or the tense muscles. The ideas and emotions racing through your head are what are causing these bodily feelings.

Beyond feelings, the mind may affect the body by

23

consciously intending to. Think about the incredible placebo effect, which demonstrates how a person's perception of getting a therapy may result in physiological changes and benefits to their health. This reveals the extraordinary impact our ideas may have on the body's capacity to heal and recover.

Intricate brain networks are also involved in the mind-body link. Through a huge network of nerves, the brain—which acts as the command center for our thoughts and actions—communicates with the body. These nerves send messages to the body that control processes including respiration, digestion, immunological response, and heart rate. The production of stress hormones like cortical, which can have a long-term impact on our health, is one of the physiological reactions that stress, for example, sets off.

On the other hand, the body and mind are profoundly interconnected. Our ideas, feelings, and general state of mind can be influenced by our physical condition. For instance, regular exercise causes the production of happy hormones like endorphins and other neurotransmitters that lessen the symptoms of sadness and anxiety. Similar to how our mood and confidence levels may be impacted by our posture and body language, research has shown that an upright posture increases emotions of empowerment and happiness.

The gut-brain connection also emphasizes the complex relationship between our digestive system and mental wellness. Our mood and cognition are significantly influenced by the gut micro biota, a complex ecology of microbes that resides there. Recent studies have highlighted the critical link between our digestive system and mental health, showing that abnormalities in the gut flora can lead to diseases like depression and anxiety.

The mind-body link may have a significant impact on our general health and quality of life, and it is something that has to be understood and used. We may learn to be aware of our thoughts, feelings, and bodily sensations by practicing mindfulness and self-awareness. We may learn to control our stress responses and improve our well-being through techniques like yoga, deep breathing, and meditation. Additionally, including physical activity in our everyday routines not only strengthens our bodies but also promotes cognitive function, emotional stability, and mental acuity. We provide our bodies with the nutrition they need for optimum mental and emotional health by eating a balanced diet.

Our ideas, emotions, bodily sensations, and general well-being are all woven together in the marvelous tapestry that is the relationship between mind and body. Each component influences and molds the others in a ballet of subtle interaction. Understanding and fostering this link gives us the capacity to live a lively and meaningful life while maximizing our health and inner potential. We open the door to releasing the power inside of us by accepting the fundamental oneness of mind and body.

Holistic Methodology for Well-Being

It takes a comprehensive approach that considers all facets of our life to achieve a sense of well-being. A thorough framework that emphasizes nourishing the body and soul to create ideal health and happiness is offered by the Holistic Methodology for Well-Being. People may promote balance and harmony in their lives by understanding the connections between these factors. This comprehensive manual presents important ideas and methods to help one live a full and fulfilled life.

The core of the holistic methodology for well-being is the body's nourishment through an appropriate diet. Emphasizing the eating of natural, whole meals gives the body the nutrients it needs for optimum performance. A balanced diet full of fruits, vegetables, whole grains, lean proteins, and healthy fats promotes physical health, increases energy, and improves general vitality. People may energize their bodies and

33

foster internal well-being by purposefully selecting healthful foods.

Physical Setting: Establishing a supportive physical setting is crucial for fostering well-being. People are encouraged by the holistic methodology to create environments that promote harmony and peace. To achieve this, living places may need to be organized and decluttered, natural components included, and spaces for rest and renewal created. People can improve their overall feeling of well-being by locating themselves in peaceful, tranquil surroundings.

Self-care as a holistic practice is a key part of the holistic methodology for well-being. It entails giving activities that support self-care and personal development a top priority. To do this, one might partake in interests, engage in self-reflection, set limits, and include relaxing techniques into everyday routines.

Making self-care a habit enables people to lower stress, boost self-esteem, and develop a positive outlook, all of which contribute to increased resilience and well-being.

The Holistic Methodology for Well-Being is a thorough and well-rounded method for nourishing the body and soul for optimum health and enjoyment. Individuals may build balance and harmony in their life by placing a high priority on a healthy diet, consistent exercise, restful sleep, fostering connections, creating a supportive physical environment, and prioritizing holistic self-care. Adopting this practice enables people to live full, diverse lives and promotes a sense of well-being that penetrates all facets of their existence.

37

Common Misconceptions about Health

Natural treatments are always secure and efficient: In recent years, interest in natural treatments and complementary therapies for a range of medical ailments has grown. It's crucial to understand that not all natural therapies are supported by scientific research and that their safety and efficacy might vary. Even while some herbal treatments have been proven to be helpful, others could interfere with pharmaceuticals or have adverse effects. Before involving any natural treatments in your treatment plan, it is crucial to speak with a doctor to be sure they are secure and appropriate for your unique illness.

The Holistic Methodology for Well-Being is a thorough and well-rounded method for nourishing the body and soul for optimum health and enjoyment. Individuals may build balance and harmony in their lives by putting a high value on a healthy diet, agreeing to exercise and restful sleep, fostering connections, creating a supportive physical environment, and prioritizing holistic self-care. Adopting this practice enables people to live diverse, full lives and promotes a sense of well-being that penetrates all facets of their existence. Natural treatments are always secure and efficient. In recent years, interest in natural treatments and complementary therapies for a range of medical ailments has grown. It is critical to recognize that not all natural remedies are backed by scientific research and that their safety and efficacy may differ. Even though some herbal treatments have been proven to be helpful, others could interfere with pharmaceuticals or have adverse effects. Before involving any natural treatments in your treatment plan, it is important to speak with a doctor to be sure they are secure and appropriate for your unique illness.

The need for and damage of vaccinations the idea that vaccinations are unneeded or even hazardous is one of the most pervasive and pernicious health myths. The development of vaccines has significantly improved public health, eliminating or significantly lowering the prevalence of several infectious illnesses, and saving countless lives. To ensure their safety, vaccines go through extensive testing. Their usefulness in avoiding illnesses and their minimal risk of side effects are confirmed by the vast body of scientific evidence. In

43

addition to placing the individual in danger, refusing vaccines contributes to the wide spread of diseases across groups that can be stopped.

All fats are unhealthy: For a long time, fats were generally demonized, which created the false impression that all fats are detrimental to your health. But not all fats are created equal. Unsaturated fats, like those in avocados, almonds, and olive oil, are advantageous to health and required by the body, in contrast to saturated and Trans fats, which are frequently found in fried meals and processed snacks.   Energy-giving, nutrient-assist,   brain-supporting,   and   skin-maintaining,   healthy   fats also help the body absorb nutrients. A well-balanced diet should include some healthy fats.

You can't work out until you're already fit: Some people   assume   that

45

exercising is only good if you are physically healthy or sporty. This myth frequently hinders people from engaging in physical exercise, resulting in a sedentary lifestyle and related health problems. Regardless of your fitness level, everyone should exercise. Numerous health advantages result from regular physical fitness, including higher mental well-being, decreased risk of chronic illnesses, increased

46

strength and flexibility, and improved cardiovascular health. Individuals of all fitness levels can incorporate exercise into their lives by beginning with low-impact exercise and progressively increasing their intensity.

Healthy food is pricey and bland: It is a frequent misperception that eating properly necessitates a major financial expenditure as well as compromising flavor and satisfaction.

While certain healthy food alternatives might be expensive, a balanced diet can be attained on a budget with careful planning and wise decisions. Fresh fruits and vegetables, complete grains, and lean meats may serve as the cornerstones of a nutritious, low-cost diet. Experimenting with herbs, spices, and other cooking techniques may also improve the flavor of nutritional meals. With a little imagination and resourcefulness, it is possible to have good and healthy cuisine without breaking the bank.

There is a misperception that mental health is less significant than physical health since physical health frequently takes center stage when talking about well-being. However, mental health is equally as important as physical health and is important for total well-being. Mental health influences how people think, feel, and act and include emotional, psychological, and social well-being. Neglecting

50

mental health can have negative effects on productivity, stress levels, and the emergence of mental diseases. It is crucial to give mental health a top priority by getting help, taking care of oneself, and having open discussions about it.

Chapter 2: Nourishing Your Body

Maintaining ideal health and fitness is more crucial than ever in our fast-paced modern society. One of the most important aspects of a healthy lifestyle is providing your body with the proper meals and minerals. We can give our bodies the vigor, vitality, and resilience they require to flourish by intentionally choosing the foods we eat. This manual intends to supply you with practical advice, perceptive knowledge, and doable methods to help your body achieve optimum health.

Understanding Nutrition's Power: Nutrition is important for maintaining our general health. It includes both the micronutrients (vitamins and minerals) and the macronutrients (carbohydrates, proteins, and fats) that our bodies need for a variety of biological processes. A balanced and diverse diet guarantees that we get enough nourishment, which promotes our best physical and mental health. The effect of healthy eating on illness prevention, lifespan, and general vigor is examined in this chapter.

Building a Healthy Plate: The key to fueling your body is building a well-balanced plate of food. The emphasis of this chapter is on including a range of whole foods in your meals. Your plate should be made up of fruits, vegetables, entire grains, lean proteins, and healthy fats. You can make conscious decisions and ensure that your meals are stocked with vital nutrients that promote overall health by being aware of portion sizes.

Portion Control and Mindful Eating: Mindful eating entails being completely present and involved in the eating

55

process. It enables us to enjoy our meals more, pay attention to our bodies' hunger and fullness cues, and create a better connection with food. The methods in this chapter can help you calm down, practice portion control, and stop eating emotionally. You may increase your pleasure in food while consuming a balanced and healthful diet by developing mindful eating habits.

Hydration for Optimal Health: Although it is important for our wellbeing, proper hydration is sometimes overlooked. Digestion, nutrition absorption, temperature control, and all other biological processes depend on water. This chapter focuses on the significance of being hydrated and provides helpful advice for improving daily water intake. It also looks at the advantages of hydrating

57

meals and drinks to keep your hydration levels at their best.

Investigating Special Dietary Considerations: Special dietary requirements, such as vegetarianism, veganism, gluten-free diets, and food allergies, require careful study to provide sufficient nutrition. These dietary options are discussed in this chapter along with their advantages and disadvantages. It provides advice on how to satisfy nutrient requirements and makes recommendations for sources of culinary inspiration and nutritional support within these dietary frameworks.

Practical Advice for Dining Out and Social Events: You don't have to forgo social gatherings or dining out if you follow a healthy diet. This chapter offers useful advice on how to choose healthier options while dining out. It offers advice on how to read restaurant menus, control portion sizes, and stick to your dietary objectives. Learn how to handle social situations, resist peer pressure, and balance enjoying social occasions with taking care of your body. Taking care of your body is a lifetime process that calls for thoughtful decision-making and persistent effort. You may enhance your health and well-being by adopting a balanced and healthy eating philosophy. You are now well-equipped to make wise judgments about what you eat thanks to the practical advice and insightful information in this extensive book. You may energize your life, feed your body, promote long-term health, and reap the rewards of a bright and active life by implementing these ideas into your daily routine. Never forget that tiny changes made now might have a big impact tomorrow. Start nourishing your body right away to experience amazing outcomes for yourself.

Balanced Nutrition

An effective diet is the cornerstone of a long and healthy life. It is the fuel that drives our bodies and supplies the crucial nutrients required for development, growth, and general health. Making thoughtful food decisions and making sure we eat a range of foods from various food categories are necessary for achieving balanced nutrition. We will examine the fundamentals of balanced nutrition in this manual and show you how to apply them to your everyday activities for optimum health.

Learning about macronutrients:

Carbohydrates, proteins, and fats are the three macronutrients that make up the majority of our diet and are the primary sources of energy. Each macronutrient has a specific function in the body and should be consumed in a balanced diet.

Carbohydrates are our main source of energy. Foods including grains, fruits, vegetables, and legumes contain them. Choose complex carbs like whole grains, which offer sustained energy and necessary fiber.

Proteins: Proteins are our bodies' building blocks and are essential for cell development and repair. Lean protein sources such as chicken, fish, beans, and nuts should be consumed. To guarantee a wide spectrum of vital amino acids, vary your protein sources.

Healthy fats: Healthy fats play an important role in hormone balance, cognitive health, and nutrition absorption. Include the monounsaturated and polyunsaturated fats that come from fatty fish, olive oil, nuts, avocados, and nuts. Reduce your intake of fried, processed, and saturated fats.

Embracing Micronutrients:

Micronutrients are the vitamins and minerals that, while being needed in lesser amounts by our bodies, are crucial for their healthy operation. **They may be**

found in a variety of foods, including:

Vitamins: To receive a variety of vitamins, eat a wide array of fruits and vegetables. Citrus fruits' vitamin C helps strengthen the immune system, while leafy greens' vitamin A supports clear vision. B vitamins help with energy metabolism and are present in whole grains and legumes.

Minerals: Include foods high in minerals in your

67

diet, such as dairy products (high in calcium), lean meats and legumes (high in iron), and nuts and seeds (high in magnesium). These minerals each support the maintenance of healthy bones, the delivery of oxygen, and the activity of enzymes.

Prioritizing Dietary Fiber: Dietary fiber is crucial for increasing satiety and preserving a healthy digestive tract. Whole grains, fruits, vegetables, legumes, and whole grains all contain it. To balance blood sugar, decrease cholesterol, and regulate bowel motions, aim for a mixture of soluble and insoluble fiber.

Hydration: A healthy diet must include water, which is frequently disregarded. Maintaining sufficient hydration assists the body's metabolism, digestion, and transportation of nutrients. Drink water often throughout the day, and

69

increase consumption when exercising or when the weather is warm.

A balanced diet is a lifetime endeavor that involves attention, understanding, and persistent effort. You may fuel your body and promote maximum health by integrating a range of macronutrients, embracing micronutrient-rich foods, emphasizing fiber, staying hydrated, exercising portion management, and creating mindful eating habits.

Remember that simple modifications in your dietary habits may have a big impact in the long run, helping you to live a more vibrant and meaningful life.

Importance of Hydration

Water, the elixir of life, is sometimes taken for granted, despite its critical role in our general health and well-being. Hydration, or providing our bodies with enough amounts of water, is critical for the proper functioning of numerous body systems. In this extensive study, we will investigate the significance of hydration and its significant influence on our bodies.

Water, which makes up around 60% of the human body, is essential for a variety of physiological functions. It acts as a structural, functional, and structurally stable component of cells, tissues, and organs. These vital systems cannot function at full capacity without enough hydration, resulting in a chain reaction of negative effects.

To begin with, hydration is critical for maintaining correct physiological fluid balance. Water serves as a vehicle for nutrients, oxygen, and hormones to go throughout the body, promoting metabolic processes and waste disposal. Adequate hydration ensures that important chemicals reach their destinations as quickly as possible, enhancing cellular processes and supporting general health. Furthermore, water is essential for maintaining body temperature. Our bodies continually seek to maintain an ideal interior temperature through a process known as thermoregulation. When we become overheated, such as during physical exertion or exposure to hot conditions, we rely on perspiration evaporation to keep us cool. Excessive sweating without replenishing fluids, on the other hand, can cause dehydration, hindering our bodies' capacity to cool down and potentially leading to heat-related disorders.

Hydration has an impact on cognitive function and mental performance as well. Mild dehydration has been demonstrated in studies to decrease cognitive capacities such as attention, memory, and focus. Inadequate hydration can cause weariness, decreased alertness, and mental clarity. As a result, being appropriately hydrated is critical for sustaining peak cognitive performance, particularly during intellectually taxing jobs, work, or study.

Hydration is important for sustaining physical health and improving general well-being, in addition to its physiological effects. Proper hydration improves digestion by improving food passage through the digestive tract and boosting nutrient absorption. It can help avoid constipation and improve regularity, ensuring that our gastrointestinal tract runs smoothly.

Furthermore, moisture is intimately related to skin health. Water is necessary for skin suppleness, dryness prevention, and promoting a youthful appearance. Well-hydrated skin is more resistant to environmental stresses, less prone to wrinkles and blemishes, and has a better complexion overall.

Hydration is a great ally for people attempting to acquire or maintain a healthy body weight. Drinking water before meals can help lower hunger and calorie consumption by creating a sensation of fullness, which aids in weight loss attempts. Furthermore, replacing water with high-calorie beverages can help reduce overall calorie consumption and avoid excessive sugar and calorie intake, resulting in a better diet and weight control.

Because of the increased fluid loss during physical activity, exercise enthusiasts and athletes, in particular, must prioritize hydration. Sweat causes significant fluid loss, which, if not supplied appropriately, can lead to dehydration, reduced performance, and an increased risk of exercise-related injury. Proper hydration is essential for boosting performance, reducing tiredness, and allowing post-workout recovery.

Ultimately, individual hydration demands vary depending on characteristics such as age, gender, exercise level, and environment. While the frequently advised suggestion of eight glasses of water per day is an excellent starting point, it is critical to listen to your body and adapt your fluid consumption appropriately. Thirst is a reliable warning that your body requires water, and it is critical to follow that signal by drinking quickly.

Finally, individual hydration demands vary depending on characteristics such as age, gender, exercise level, and environment. While the frequently advised suggestion of eight glasses of water per day is an excellent starting point, it is critical to listen to your body and adapt your fluid consumption appropriately. Thirst is a reliable warning that your body requires water, and it is critical to follow that signal by drinking quickly.

Mindful Eating

We frequently eat more while we are multitasking while eating, whether it be working through lunch or watching TV while eating dinner. On the other hand, eating "mindfully," or taking time to appreciate each bite, improves the dining experience and keeps us conscious of how much we consume.

Meals have become just another daily activity we cram in thanks to our fast-food culture. It is all too typical to hear about individuals getting breakfast on the go or attending a lunch meeting where business is the main focus and eating is only the enticement to get folks there.

Adults in the United States eat for an average of 1 hour and 12 minutes each day, yet watch television for between 212 and 3 hours every day. Our children are also pressed for time. According to studies, school lunch periods offer pupils an average of 7 to 11 minutes to eat their meal. There are more issues besides just how quickly we eat. We frequently combine eating with other activities like driving or working at our desks since we are a nation of multitaskers. We don't often just eat when we're eating. In actuality, 66% of Americans say they frequently eat dinner in front of the TV. Given the pandemic levels of obesity,

85

we must examine how we eat as well as what we eat.

The Effects of Mindful Eating

It may come as a surprise to hear that "mindless" eating, or eating without consciousness, can be harmful to one's health. Scientists are starting to assess and comprehend the intricate function of the mind-body relationship in eating behavior. It turns out that when we shut out our minds during meals, the digestion process is 30% to 40% less effective. This can lead to digestive issues including gas, bloating, and bowel irregularities.

Aside from gas and bloating, overeating and obesity are two of the most serious health issues induced, at least in part, by thoughtless eating. The mind-body link is critical to our capacity to correctly judge hunger and fullness.

87

While the exact mechanics of hunger and fullness are unknown, we do know that the brain and central nervous system receive signals from the body when food is sought or required. Many factors, including psychological states such as our emotions, might elicit these signals.

When eating begins, the brain plays an important role in sending a signal that fullness is near. Critical signals that govern food intake may be missed if the mind is "multi-tasking" while eating. If the brain does not receive some messages that occur during eating, such as taste sensation and enjoyment, the experience may not be registered as "eating." This circumstance may cause the brain to continue sending out hunger signals, raising the likelihood of overeating.

How to Practice Eating Mindfully

89

Mindful eating entails eating with mindfulness. Not awareness of the things on your plate, but rather awareness of the dining experience. Mindful eating entails being present for each sensation that arises during eating, such as chewing, tasting, and swallowing, moment by moment. If you've ever tried to practice mindfulness in any form (such as meditation, relaxation, or breathing exercises), you know how quickly our thoughts may stray. When we eat, the same thing happens. When you first start practicing mindful eating, remember not to condemn yourself if you catch your thoughts wandering away from the sensation of eating. Instead, simply return to the knowledge of that taste while you chew, bite, or swallow. Try the following activity if this topic is new to you.

Mindful eating entails eating with mindfulness. Not awareness of the things on your plate, but rather awareness of the dining experience. Mindful eating is being present for each sensation that arises throughout the eating process, such as chewing, tasting, and swallowing, moment by moment. If you've ever tried to practice mindfulness in any form (such as meditation, relaxation, or breathing exercises), you know how quickly our thoughts may stray. When we eat, the same thing happens. When you first start practicing mindful eating, remember not to condemn yourself if you catch your thoughts wandering away from the sensation of eating. Instead, simply return to the knowledge of that taste while you chew, bite, or swallow.

93

Try the following activity if this topic is new to you: Perform this activity with a friend. Each individual will require one little piece of an apple. While one person reads the directions below, the other person completes the activity.

Close your eyes after taking one bite of an apple slice. Do not start chewing quite yet.

Try not to think about the thoughts that are racing through your head; instead,

94

concentrate on the apple. Take note of anything that comes to mind regarding flavor, texture, warmth, and sensations in your mouth. Begin chewing right away. Chew carefully, only noting how it feels. It's natural for your thoughts to stray. If you feel yourself paying more attention to your thoughts than to your chewing, simply let the notion go for a second and return your concentration to the chewing. Take note of

95

every single movement of your jaw.

You might wish to consume the apple during these times. Try to stay focused and note the tiny shift from chewing to swallowing.

Try to follow the apple as it moves toward the back of your tongue and into your throat as you prepare to swallow it. Swallow the apple, following it until you can no longer feel any food feeling.

Exhale after taking a long breath.

You might find it fascinating to discuss your experience with your partner. What did you observe while you chewed? What made you swallow? Was the food no longer appetizing? Did it disintegrate? Were you uninterested?

The purpose of this exercise is not to propose that you consume all of your meals as methodically as in this trial. Rather, by participating in this activity, you may learn something about your eating patterns. Some individuals believe that completing a shorter version of this exercise with the first bite of each meal is beneficial. This helps to set the goal of being aware during your meal. Here are a few more ideas for incorporating mindfulness into eating. Try them out and see what you come up with!

Simple starting steps to incorporating mindfulness when eating:

Use chopsticks to eat.
Use your non-dominant hand to eat.
Chew your meal between 30 and 50 times per bite.
Eat without watching TV, reading the newspaper, or using a computer.
Eat when seated.

Put enough food on your plate and attempt to make the meal last at least 20 minutes.

The Role of Supplements

Supplements have grown in popularity in recent years as individuals attempt to improve their health and well-being. These supplements, which range from vitamins and minerals to herbal extracts and specialty chemicals, are intended to supplement a healthy diet and address nutritional deficiencies. In this in-depth examination, we will look at the function of supplements in maintaining a healthy lifestyle and how they may be used to improve general well-being.

Bridging Nutritional Disparities

While a well-balanced diet is the cornerstone of good health, it is difficult to receive all the elements needed from food alone. Modern diets frequently lack certain vitamins, minerals, and other essential components as a result of factors such as hectic lives, poor dietary choices, and food processing processes. Supplements serve as a bridge, ensuring that we acquire the essential elements that our diets may be lacking. They can aid in the maintenance of normal body functioning, immunological health, and energy levels.

Supporting Specific Health Objectives

Supplements are not one-size-fits-all: instead, they may be customized to fulfill individual health objectives. Athletes, for example, regularly utilize protein supplements to aid with muscle repair and growth. Omega-3 fatty acid supplements are popular due to their possible cardiovascular and cognitive advantages. Pregnant mothers may use folic acid supplements to protect their newborns against neural tube abnormalities. The beauty of supplements is their adaptability, which allows individuals to efficiently meet their health demands.

Considering Lifestyle Factors.

Our lifestyle choices may have an impact on our nutritional status. Individuals following strict vegetarian or vegan diets, for example, may struggle to receive enough vitamin B12, which is predominantly found in animal sources. Supplements can help compensate for these dietary restrictions by ensuring that essential nutrients are not missed.

Advocating for Age-Related Changes

Our nutritional requirements fluctuate as we age. It may be difficult for older persons to ingest enough calcium to maintain bone health or vitamin D to help in calcium absorption. Supplements designed specifically for the requirements of aging people can provide a solution by increasing bone strength, cognitive function, and immunological support in the later stages of life.

Filling Nutritional Gaps During Stressful Times

Stressful times in life, such as illness or strenuous physical exercise, can raise the body's dietary requirements. Supplements can be quite beneficial in boosting the body's immune system and healing processes during these periods. Vitamin C, zinc, and elderberry supplements, for example, are known to have immune-boosting characteristics that can help the body fight off infections and recover more quickly.

Micronutrient Deficiency Correction

107

Individuals may develop micronutrient shortages in some situations owing to underlying health concerns, malabsorption disorders, or limited diets. Healthcare providers can prescribe supplements to help rectify these deficits and enhance general health. Regular nutrition level monitoring is required to successfully identify and rectify such shortages.

Increasing Exercise Performance

Certain supplements can improve workout performance and help with muscle recovery for fitness lovers. Creatine supplements, for example, are well-known for their potential to enhance energy levels during high-intensity exercises, whilst branched-chain amino acids (BCAAs) can help minimize exercise-induced muscle damage and soreness.

Antioxidant and anti-inflammatory support

Many supplements have antioxidant and anti-inflammatory characteristics that can assist the body in a variety of ways. Antioxidants help neutralize damaging free radicals, protecting cells from oxidative stress and lowering the risk of chronic illnesses. Turmeric and curcumin supplements, for example, are recognized for their significant anti-inflammatory properties, which may aid those suffering from illnesses such as arthritis.

Maintaining Good Mental Health

The gut-brain link has gained popularity in recent years. Certain supplements, such as probiotics and prebiotics, have been shown to improve gut health, perhaps leading to mental well-being advantages. Furthermore, omega-3 fatty acid supplementation, such as fish oil, has been linked to enhanced mood and cognitive performance.

Helping Digestion and Gut Health

Digestive enzymes and fiber supplements can assist to enhance digestion and gut health. Individuals suffering from digestive problems such as irritable bowel syndrome (IBS) or lactose intolerance may benefit from these supplements.

Supplements provide a variety of health advantages, from bridging dietary deficiencies to supporting particular health objectives and treating age-related changes or lifestyle issues.

Supplements can improve overall health and quality of life when taken appropriately and in conjunction with a balanced diet. However, it is critical to speak with a healthcare practitioner before beginning any supplement program, as individual requirements and potential interactions with drugs must be considered. Adopting a holistic approach to health that includes a well-balanced diet, frequent exercise, and

suitable supplements can
pave the way for a better,
happier life.

Chapter 3: Moving and Exercising

A Path to a Healthier, Happier You Embrace the Joy of Movement: Whether it's dancing to your favorite music, taking leisurely walks in nature, practicing yoga for flexibility and mindfulness, or participating in recreational sports with friends, finding activities that resonate with you can make incorporating movement into your daily routine a delightful experience.

Understand Exercise Science: Science demonstrates the remarkable advantages of exercise for our general health. Regular exercise not only builds our muscles and bones but also enhances our immune system, cardiovascular health, and length of life. On a mental level, exercise encourages the production of endorphins, which increase mood and lower stress, resulting in greater mental health and improved cognitive performance.

Unleash Your Inner Athlete: Everyone possesses an athlete inside them just waiting to be released. Set objectives and push yourself to reach new heights. To notice development and improvements, gradually increase your workout's time and intensity. The sense of satisfaction you get from overcoming new obstacles will increase your confidence and motivate you to keep pushing yourself.

The Power of Consistency: The secret to maximizing the benefits of moving and working out is consistency. Instead of seeing exercise as a one-time thing, make it a habit. Even if you have to start off with only a few minutes every day, make a realistic timetable and adhere to it. Your body and mind will eventually adjust, and you'll start to want those endorphins and the energizing sensation that comes after each workout.

Fun and Social Connection: Working out doesn't have to be a solitary activity. Make it a social experience by inviting friends, family, or joining a fitness club. Social support may help with accountability, inspiration, and enjoyment of the path toward a healthy way of life. Consistency is important, but so is understanding your body's messages. Not only is exercise important, but so is relaxation and recovery. Pay attention to any pain or indications of exhaustion, and give your body the time it requires to heal and regenerate.

You may alter yourself by moving and working out. Remember to treasure the thrill of movement, respect the science behind your efforts, and embrace the potent link between mind and body as you set out on your road to a healthier, happier self. Maintain consistency, make attainable goals, and, most importantly, take pleasure in the journey. Let exercise be the means to a more contented and energetic life, and let movement be your celebration of life. Accept the power of movement and exercise, and observe how it improves every aspect of your life!

Finding Joy in Physical Activity

Finding enjoyment in physical activity is not only good but essential for our general well-being in today's fast-paced world when stress and sedentary lives have become the norm. Regular exercise has a significant influence on our mental and emotional health in addition to improving our physical health. Accepting physical exercise may help us find new levels of happiness, pleasure, and energy. We'll explore the many ways physical activity may make your life happier and more exciting in this investigation.

Release Endorphin Power: Endorphins, or the "feel-good" hormones, are released in response to physical exertion. Your body manufactures these organic mood enhancers when you work out, leaving you feeling euphoric and content. Endorphins perform their magic when you feel that post-workout glow and the uplifted feeling that goes along with it. Your training regimen may become a fun adventure thanks to the endorphin surge, which can be experienced when dancing, running, swimming, or cycling.

Embark on experiences:
Exercise allows you to embark on a variety of experiences. Step outside of the boundaries of your routine and enjoy nature. Explore beautiful woods on foot, scale imposing mountains, or simply stroll along the shore. Adventure activities like rock climbing, kayaking, or surfing give you a sense of success and adrenaline while also leaving you with priceless memories

that will make you happy for years to come.

Accept the Mind-Body Connection: A key component of finding joy in physical activity is developing a deeper connection with your body. Excellent exercises that encourage mindfulness and self-awareness include yoga, tai chi, and pilates. You'll feel quiet and tranquillity as you pay attention to your breath, stretch, and move elegantly. This mindful kind

127

of exercise cultivates a healthy relationship between your mind and body, producing a profound sense of joy and well-being.

Join a Community: Working out doesn't have to be something you do alone. Joining a running club, sports team, or fitness class gives you access to a supportive group of people who share your interests. Shared objectives, encouragement, and companionship build a social connection that improves your life. A hard workout may become a pleasant group activity when done with others, making the process much more pleasurable and fulfilling.

Celebrate Your Progress, Not Perfection: Embracing physical exercise is about recognizing your progress and effort, not about obtaining perfection. Set attainable objectives and celebrate your progress along the way. Every success, whether it be learning a new workout or building your stamina, makes you feel proud and happy. Keep in mind that the joy of the journey itself, not how far you've gone, is what matters.

Identify Your Passion: There are many different types of physical activity. Try out different things to see which ones most appeal to you. You could fall in love with dancing, weightlifting, or participating in a team sport. Accept the thrill of trying out many pursuits until you discover your passion. Physical activity becomes less of a duty and more of an enjoyable experience when you are doing something you truly like.

We may access a source of happiness and well-being that can have a positive effect on every element of our being by embracing physical exercise and implementing it into our daily lives. Physical activity offers a route to a happier and healthier self, from the euphoric surge of endorphins to the quiet of mindfulness and the sense of success within a community. So put on your running shoes, grab your yoga mat, or go on your bike and immerse yourself in the pleasures of physical activity to live a more vital and contented life.

Types of Exercise for Different Goals

Loss of Weight: Running, jogging, cycling, jumping rope, and swimming are examples of cardiovascular exercises.

High-Intensity Interval Training (HIIT): Rapid-fire bouts of vigorous exercise interspersed with quick rests.

Circuit training: A series of quick strength and cardiovascular workouts.

133

Dancing: Exercises like Zumba, hip-hop, and other dancing forms are enjoyable ways to burn calories.

Aerobics: Regular, rhythmic exercises are used in traditional aerobics sessions.

Weightlifting, or compound workouts like squats, deadlifts, bench presses, and overhead presses, is a good way to build muscle (hypertrophy).

134

Bodyweight exercises include lunges, dips, push-ups, and bodyweight squats. Utilizing resistance bands or equipment to focus on certain muscle areas is known as resistance training.

Isolation Exercises: Concentrating on certain muscles, such as tricep extensions and bicep curls. Strength and Power: Powerlifting: Using heavy weights to compete in bench press, squat, and deadlift competitions.

Olympic weightlifting: Develop explosive power with lifts like the clean and jerk and snatch.

Plyometrics: Spontaneous exercises include depth leaps, medicine ball tosses, and box jumps.

Kettlebell Training: Making use of kettlebell workouts to increase power and strength. Mobility and **Flexibility:**

Yoga: Through a variety of positions and stretches, you may increase your flexibility, balance, and core strength.

Pilates: A set of exercises meant to enhance posture, flexibility, and strength.

Dynamic stretching: To increase range of motion, stretching exercises are combined with movement.

Foam rolling: Making use of a foam roller to alleviate tension in the muscles and increase mobility.

General health and stamina:

Brisk Walking: A straightforward and efficient low-impact workout for general fitness and health.

Cycling: Using a stationary bike or an outdoor cycle to increase endurance.

Swimming: A low-impact, all-over-body exercise that strengthens the heart.

Hiking: Appreciating the outdoors while testing physical stamina and strength on various terrains.

Mind-body connection and stress reduction

Tai Chi: A mild martial technique that emphasizes flexibility, balance, and meditation.

Mindfulness Meditation: Using mindfulness and relaxation methods to improve one's mental health.

Qigong: A mind-body exercise that includes rhythmic motions and deep breathing.

Nature Walks: Spending time outside might help you feel calmer and think more clearly.

To be sure the exercises are appropriate for your unique requirements and skills, always speak with a healthcare expert or a licensed fitness trainer before beginning any exercise program.

Incorporating Movement into Daily Life

For one to maintain a healthy lifestyle, activity must be included in everyday life. The effects of inactivity on one's physical and mental health can be detrimental. Here are some helpful hints to help you include exercise in your daily activities:

Take the steps: Whenever possible, choose the steps over the elevator or escalator. A great technique to work your legs and get your heart rate up is to climb stairs.

Consider riding a bike or walking to work if it's an option. Not only is it a great way to get some exercise, but it also lowers carbon emissions and traffic jams.

Active Commuting: If your employment is far away, consider parking further away or taking public transit and getting off one or two stops earlier so you may walk the remaining distance.

Lunchtime Walks: Take advantage of your lunch hour by going for a quick stroll. You can unwind and renew your thoughts with this exercise, which will help you have a productive day.

Regularly stand up: Whether you're at home or at work, make it a point to stand up every hour or so. To prevent prolonged sitting, provide reminders if necessary.

Desk activities: To relieve stiffness and boost

circulation, perform quick exercises at your desk, including stretching, leg lifts, and shoulder rolls.

Active Meetings: If appropriate, think about holding meetings outside with your coworkers. You may talk about things while exercising and enjoying the outdoors.

Domestic tasks: Take advantage of the chance to move by embracing domestic tasks. Physical exercise is required for vacuuming, cleaning, gardening, and even cooking.

Play some music and dance or move around while performing everyday duties or in your free time. It's a good way to get moving and improve your attitude.

Make use of games and applications for fitness that promote physical exercise. These applications frequently provide incentives and challenges, which add interest to exercise.

Stretching before bed: Before going to sleep, do some light stretching. It may aid in muscular relaxation and improve sleep.

When running errands or shopping, park further away from the entrance to give oneself more space to go around on foot.

Family Activities: Take part in physical activities such as sports, walks, or picnics in the park with your family or friends.

Take Breaks While Watching TV: Use commercial breaks during TV or movie viewing sessions to perform brief workouts or stretches.

Discover New Interests: Take up a new activity that requires mobility, such as dance, yoga, or martial arts. These pursuits can improve your health while also being pleasant.

Always look for opportunities to exercise and stay active throughout the day. You may improve your general well-being and make exercise an effortless and necessary part of your routine by introducing movement into your everyday life.

Overcoming Barriers to Exercise

The key to maintaining a healthy lifestyle and

attaining fitness objectives is removing obstacles to exercising. There are several barriers that people must overcome to engage in regular physical activity. One's capacity to fit exercise into their daily schedule can be greatly improved by recognizing and removing these obstacles. **The following are some typical obstacles to exercise and solutions to them:**

Lack of Time: In the busy world we live in today, finding time to exercise might be difficult. Consider adding physical activity to your regular agenda to get over this obstacle. Exercises that are brief and intensive, or even 15 to 30 minutes of brisk walking, can be helpful. If you can't find a block of free time, attempt to spread out your workout into smaller periods throughout the day.

Lack of drive: Maintaining consistent exercise motivation can be challenging, especially when establishing a new habit. Setting clear, doable objectives and monitoring your progress are two ways to overcome this obstacle. Finding a workout partner or enrolling in a fitness class may also help you be accountable and supported, which will help you stay motivated.

151

Physical restrictions or health problems: Some medical illnesses or physical restrictions might make performing traditional exercise difficult. Before beginning any new fitness regimen, you must speak with a healthcare provider. They may assist in creating a training regimen that fits your unique requirements and capabilities.

Fear of Injury: For some people, exercising because they are afraid of being wounded might be quite difficult. Start with low-impact exercises that are easier on the body, like yoga, cycling, or swimming, to address this worry. Injury risk can also be decreased by adopting the right workout routines, warm-ups, and cool-downs.

Lack of Social Support: Support from friends, family, or the fitness community may significantly help. Participating in group activities or discussing your workout experience with others may offer support, accountability, and friendship.

Financial Restrictions:
Specialized equipment, workout classes, and gym memberships can be pricey. But getting in shape doesn't have to be expensive. Running and bodyweight workouts are two inexpensive choices that need little to no equipment. Extreme weather or a lack of access to safe exercise areas might prevent people from engaging in outdoor activities. Having a backup indoor plan, such as

155

exercising at home, watching exercise videos, or visiting indoor facilities, will help you get through this obstacle.

Lack of knowledge: People may be deterred from attempting if they don't know where to begin or how to exercise effectively. It might be helpful to seek advice from fitness experts, such as personal trainers or exercise apps, as they can offer individualized workout regimens and useful information.

Job-Life Balance: Making time for fitness while juggling a job, family, and personal obligations can be challenging. A better work-life-exercise balance may be achieved by prioritizing and planning physical activity as part of your daily schedule.

Unrealistic Expectations: Having unrealistic expectations while setting exercise objectives might make you feel frustrated and disappointed. To keep motivated, set small, attainable goals at first and recognize your progress.

People may make exercise a pleasant and lasting part of their life and enhance their physical and emotional well-being by recognizing these barriers and using workable solutions to get through them.

Getting enough rest and sleep is crucial to leading a balanced, healthy lifestyle. Both are essential for fostering both physical and mental well-being. Here are some crucial ideas regarding rest and sleep:

Rest: Rest is important because it gives the body and mind time to repair and regenerate after exerting themselves physically or mentally.

Sorts of Rest: There are many different sorts of rest, including social rest (taking a break from social contacts), emotional rest (lowering stress and emotional strain), mental rest (relaxing the mind), and physical rest (resting the body).

Advantages of Sleep: A good night's sleep lowers stress levels, enhances cognitive performance, increases productivity, and improves general health and well-being.

Work-Life Balance: To avoid burnout and maintain a healthy lifestyle, it's important to strike a balance between work, leisure time, and rest.

Short afternoon naps might help recharge batteries and improve attentiveness throughout the day.

Sleep: Sleep is a natural condition of rest for the body and mind and is important for maintaining physical and mental health as well as cognitive and emotional well-being.

Rapid Eye Movement (REM) and Non-Rapid Eye Movement (NREM) sleep are two sleep cycles that each have their own functions to perform during the sleep cycle.

Recommended Sleep Duration: Adults need, on average, 7-9 hours of sleep each night to perform at their best. The quantity of

163

sleep required changes with age.

Sleep and Memory Consolidation: The brain absorbs information learned throughout the day and consolidates memories when we sleep, which helps us learn and retain knowledge.

Insomnia hygiene Creating a sleep-friendly atmosphere, keeping a regular sleep schedule, and minimizing screen time before bedtime are all ways to enhance sleep quality.

Advice for More Restful Sleep:

To tell your body it's time to wind down and get ready for bed, establish a soothing evening ritual.

To encourage improved sleep quality, make sure your sleeping environment is cozy, peaceful, and dark.

Avoid consuming large meals, coffee, and electronics just before bed

165

since these things might disturb your sleep cycle.

Regular exercise can enhance sleep, but avoid strenuous exercises right before bed.

Use relaxation techniques to ease stress, such as meditation or deep breathing exercises.

Remember that everyone has different demands for rest and sleep, so it's important to pay attention to your body and modify your schedule as necessary to have the greatest possible rest and sleep.

Understanding the Importance of Rest

It's essential to comprehend the value of rest if you want to preserve general well-being and increase productivity. Rest may take many different forms, including physical, mental, and sleep. People frequently disregard the value of rest in today's fast-paced and demanding society, which has several detrimental effects. Consider the following significant factors: **Physical Recuperation:** Sleep is crucial for our bodies' recuperation and renewal. Our bodies go through important activities when we sleep, including hormone control, muscular development, and tissue repair. Physical weariness, reduced immune systems, and greater susceptibility to infections can all result from insufficient sleep.

Mental Clarity and Focus: Our minds need downtime to operate at their best, just as our bodies do. Without pauses, continuous cognitive exertion can result in burnout, decreased attention, and poor decision-making. Taking pauses while working or studying can boost creativity and productivity.

Reduction of Stress: Sleep is essential for stress

management. Our bodies release chemicals during sleep that work to balance out stress hormones and encourage relaxation. On the other side, persistent stress can result in anxiety, sadness, and a variety of physical health problems.

Improved Learning and Memory: Rest, especially sleep, is essential for learning and memory consolidation. The brain organizes and integrates daytime data during deep sleep cycles, which makes it simpler to recall and retain information.

Rest can improve one's capacity for both creativity and problem-solving. The mind may form new connections and come up with novel answers when the body is given a respite from a challenging endeavor.

Physical and mental well-being: Chronic sleep loss and insufficient rest are linked to many health

171

difficulties, including heart disease, obesity, diabetes, and mental health conditions like sadness and anxiety.

Balanced Life: Making sleep a priority promotes better work-life harmony. It helps us to schedule time for activities such as work, relationships, leisure, and self-care, resulting in a life that is more gratifying and meaningful.

Longevity: Research has shown that those who value

sleep and relaxation tend to be healthier in the long run and may even live longer.

Performance: Athletes in particular are aware of the value of rest for enhancing performance. For muscle regeneration, injury prevention, and optimal performance, proper rest and recovery are crucial. Knowing the value of sleep extends beyond realizing its significance in preventing burnout. Rest is an essential component of human

173

functioning that affects one's physical well-being, mental clarity, and level of happiness in life as a whole. Our lives may be healthier, more successful, and more meaningful if we prioritize sleep.

Establishing Healthy Sleep Habits

For sustaining total well-being and ensuring the best possible physical and mental health, it is essential to establish appropriate sleeping habits, commonly referred to as excellent sleep hygiene. Our bodies may relax, mend, and revitalize via sleep, a vital biological activity. Lack of sleep can cause a variety of health problems, such as immune system deterioration, mood swings, and cognitive impairment.

Here are some crucial pointers to help you develop healthy sleeping habits:

175

Consistent Sleep Schedule: Even on weekends, try to go to bed and wake up at the same times every day. This encourages better-quality sleep by regulating your body's internal schedule.

Establish a peaceful Pre-Sleep habit: Set up a peaceful pre-sleep habit that tells your body it's time to relax. This can entail doing something relaxing like reading a book, having a warm bath, or engaging in deep breathing exercises or meditation.

Limit Caffeine and Stimulants: Caffeine, nicotine, and other stimulants shouldn't be used right before bedtime since they might interfere with your ability to get to sleep and stay asleep.

Create a Sleep-Conducive Environment: Make sure your bedroom is cozy and sleep-friendly. Maintain a cool, calm environment in the room, and spend money on a cozy mattress and pillows.

Limit Your Screen Time: Blue light from electronics like computers, cellphones, and tablets can keep you from falling asleep. At least an hour before going to bed, try to reduce screen time.

Regular physical activity can improve sleep quality, but avoid strenuous activity right before bed since it could interfere with falling asleep.

Watch Your Diet: Pay attention to what you consume, particularly in the evening. Spicy foods, large meals, and a lot of liquids right before bed can all interfere with your sleep.

Manage Stress: Anxiety and stress can interfere with sleep. Engage in stress-relieving activities like yoga, mindfulness, or enjoyable hobbies.

Limit Daytime Napping: While taking naps throughout the day might

179

be beneficial, doing so too frequently or too close to bedtime can disrupt nocturnal sleep.

Limit Alcohol: While alcohol may initially make you feel sleepy, it can alter sleep cycles and result in less restful sleep.

Seek Natural Light Exposure: Spending time outside during the day can help you get enough natural light to improve your body's sleep-wake cycle.

Avoid monitoring the clock Constantly: Constantly monitoring the clock while in bed might heighten sleep anxiety and make it harder to fall asleep. Individual sleep requirements might vary, so it's important to pay attention to your body and modify it as necessary. If you frequently have trouble sleeping despite developing healthy sleep habits, think about speaking with a healthcare provider or sleep expert to determine and treat any underlying sleep disorders or difficulties. The basis of general health and well-being is quality sleep, so investing in good sleep habits can pay off in the long run.

Managing Stress for Better Sleep

To sleep better, stress has to be well managed. Our bodies release chemicals like cortisol and adrenaline in

response to stress, which can interfere with our regular sleep-wake cycle and make it difficult to get to sleep or stay asleep. Chronic stress can cause sleep apnea and even insomnia in the long run. **However, there are many techniques you may use to successfully manage stress and encourage better sleep:**
Establish a Regular Sleep Schedule: Attempt to go to bed and rise at the same times every day, including

183

on weekends. This enhances the general effectiveness of your sleep and assists in regulating your body's internal clock.

Establish a Calming Bedtime Habit: Before going to bed, establish a tranquil habit to let your body know that it's time to unwind. Reading a book, having a warm bath, or engaging in relaxation techniques can all help to lower tension and encourage better sleep.

Limit Your Exposure to Electronics: The blue light emitted by smartphones, tablets, and laptops might prevent the body from producing melatonin, which is essential for sleep. To get better quality sleep, try to avoid screens for at least an hour before bed.

Regular Physical Activity: Physical activity regularly can assist lower stress levels and improve sleep. However, avoid doing a strenuous workout just

185

before bed because it could make it harder to fall asleep. Identify the sources of your stress and make an effort to control them throughout the day. This may entail time management, setting limits, asking friends and family for support, or even seeking professional assistance through counseling or therapy.

Power of Relaxation Techniques

Real relaxation might seem like an unattainable dream due to the stress of contemporary life. However, there is no need for tension and worry to rule your life. You may easily recover the joy in life if you take the time to study the art of relaxing. A regulated state of mind is the key to relaxing. You may, for instance, spend an

187

entire hour in a spa, but how can you unwind if you are always thinking about the future?

Restorative Practices

The Present Is All That Matters: How frequently do we find ourselves fretting about the future? A large percentage of our thoughts are consumed with worry about the future. To be honest, though, thinking about the future does nothing to help. You will never be able to unwind if

188

you constantly dwell on the past or the future. Living just in the present moment is what it means to be relaxed.

Your surroundings matter: Where you spend your time has a slight impact on how you feel. Although we may not always be conscious of it, you'll notice that some spaces make it simpler to unwind and find serenity.

Look around your room: if there are any messes, they

189

will serve as continual reminders of what has to be done.

These persistent internal reminders weigh heavily on the psyche. You'll feel much better and be able to relax if you organize the space and make it a nice place to be. Don't be afraid to spend a little money on items like flowers and air fresheners. Spend some time organizing your living and working spaces.

It's necessary for relaxation and will increase your productivity.

Meditation: During meditation, we deliberately set aside time to quiet the mind and emphasize a genuine sense of calm. Meditation is beneficial because it teaches us how to manage our thoughts' constant stream. The goal of meditation is to maintain mental stillness, which promotes clarity and inner tranquility. The finest kind

191

of relaxation is when we are liberated from the unending cares and fears we have created for ourselves. Spend 10 or 15 minutes each day in meditation; this will help you effortlessly distance yourself from the stresses of the outside world.

Productivity not **Procrastination:** Relaxation does not include lying on a beach all day. Even in the thick of our everyday duties, we must learn to unwind. Set priorities for the tasks you have to do. You'll feel less pressured and complete tasks faster if you approach them methodically and one at a time. We put ourselves under a lot of pressure when we attempt to perform numerous things at once, and it is this battle that prevents us from being able to unwind. Avoid making things difficult for yourself. Focus on one item at a time and have fun with it. When all the essential labor has been done, the reward is being able to enjoy yourself guilt-free.

Don't Rely on Others' Opinions: To what extent do you rely on the opinions of others? We put stress on our minds when we are concerned about what other people might think or say. We strive unconsciously to appease other people. However, it is hard to unwind when we are in this frame of mind. There will always be someone who tries to criticize or find fault with anything we do or say. As a result, we should practice being detached from both praise and criticism.

This doesn't imply that we don't care about what other people think; it only means that we won't let their beliefs lead us to lose our inner calm. Although we may gradually assign less weight to other people's opinions over time, this piece of advice is difficult to put into practice. Only

195

when we stop thinking about what others are saying and doing can we truly relax?

Make Time for Yourself: Don't let work or other people dictate your schedule all the time; schedule some time just for you. Take evasive action if you are receiving frequent phone calls and emails that are harassing. Only respond to emails and phone calls during specific hours of the day. It's doubtful that having you available at all times is necessary. Relaxation becomes quite difficult when we let stress mount. You should be able to lessen the demands made on your time and energy, though, if you work extremely hard at it.

A change is as nice as a rest: Life shouldn't be a serialized soap opera that never ends. Do something radically different if you sense yourself becoming stale in your routine. For instance,

197

you won't feel truly relaxed if you spend your nights watching pointless TV or surfing the internet. Take a stroll or engage in some exercise. You'll be able to unwind and escape the monotony and aggravation of everyday activity with the change of scenery and exercise.

Gentle breathing is all it takes to relax.

Take a break if you're feeling anxious. Observe and be conscious of your breathing. Natural, gentle breathing will have a very strong, relaxing effect on your thoughts. Feel as though you are inhaling inner serenity as you inhale. Feel as though you are expelling all of your concerns and fears when you exhale. Relaxation doesn't have to be difficult at all; it can be this simple.

Chapter 5: Building Mental and Emotional Health

For general well-being and coping with adversity in life, developing mental and emotional health is essential. The following techniques and tactics can support physical, mental, and emotional health:

Practice mindfulness: Mindfulness entails paying full attention to the present moment and monitoring thoughts and feelings without passing judgment. Stress, worry, and unfavorable thought patterns can all be lessened with its aid.

Exercise frequently: Endorphins, which naturally elevate mood are released through physical exercise. Exercise regularly can assist with stress management, better sleep, and self-esteem.

Healthy Eating: Consuming a variety of

fruits, vegetables, healthy grains, and lean meats helps maintain emotional stability and nourishes the brain with critical nutrients.

Make getting adequate sleep each night a priority. For cognitive performance, emotional control, and general mental wellness, sleep is essential.

Social Connections: Develop and preserve wholesome friendships and family ties. In times of stress, social support is essential and can strengthen a sense of identity and purpose.

Set attainable objectives by breaking down larger ones into more manageable chunks. This strategy can boost motivation while reducing feelings of overload.

Seek Professional Assistance: Don't be afraid to contact a mental health professional if you are experiencing mental or emotional difficulties.

203

Counseling and therapy can offer important support and direction.

Practice Gratitude: Regularly set aside time to think about what you have to be thankful for. Positive attitudes may be fostered and bad thoughts can be diverted by feeling grateful.

Limit Stress: Identify the sources of your stress and develop coping mechanisms for them. Setting limits, managing your time, or getting help may be necessary for this.

Hobbies: Take part in pursuits that make you happy and fulfilled. Hobbies can help you feel more accomplished and can be a way to relieve stress.

Limit Screen Time: Limit your use of social media and electronic gadgets, which can have a negative influence on your mental health and interfere with your sleep.

Practice Self-Compassion: Be nice and understanding to yourself just as you would be to a friend. When things are tough, be gentle to yourself. Volunteering and providing assistance to others can improve moods and foster a sense of fulfillment and purpose.

Limit Substance Use: Restrict alcohol and drug intake to avoid damaging effects on mental and emotional stability.

206

Develop Resilience:
Although life can be unpleasant at times, being resilient can help you recover from setbacks and cope with hard circumstances.

Keep in mind that improving your mental and emotional health takes time, so it's acceptable to ask for help and take baby steps in the right direction. Be gentle to yourself and congratulate yourself on your successes as they happen.

207

Building Resilience

Imagine that you are going on a river rafting expedition. Your chart indicates that in addition to sluggish water and shallow areas, you will experience inescapable rapids and curves. How would you ensure that you can successfully navigate the choppy waters and deal with any unanticipated issues that arise from the challenge?

You could ask more seasoned travelers for advice while you plan your route or count on the company of reliable friends while traveling. Perhaps you would bring an additional life jacket or think about **Employing a more powerful raft. One thing is certain:** With the appropriate equipment and assistance, you won't only survive the difficulties of your river expedition. You'll

209

grow more fearless and confident as a result.

Describe resilience.

Everyone will face twists and turns in life, from routine difficulties to horrific incidents with longer-lasting effects, such as the loss of a loved one, a life-changing accident, or a major disease. Life may not come with a map. Every shift has a varied impact on individuals, bringing with it a distinct onslaught of ideas, potent emotions, and uncertainty.   However, resilience plays a key role in how successfully people adjust over time to stressful and life-changing experiences.

Resilience is the ability to adapt successfully in the face of adversity, trauma, tragedy, danger, or severe causes of stress, such as issues with family and relationships, serious health issues, or challenges in the financial and professional spheres. Resilience may result in significant personal improvement in addition to just "bouncing back" from these trying events.

While these unfortunate occurrences are undoubtedly painful and challenging, similar to choppy river waves, they don't have to decide how your life turns out. There are numerous facets of your life that you can manage, change, and develop. That is resilience's function.

Gaining greater resiliency

not only enables you to overcome challenging situations but also gives you the capacity to develop and even enhance your life.

What Resilience isn't

Being resilient does not guarantee that a person won't face challenges or go through difficult times. Emotional anguish and stress are frequently experienced by those who have experienced significant difficulty or tragedy in their lives. The path to resilience is likely to require a great deal of emotional pain.

While certain circumstances may make some people more resilient than others, resilience isn't always a quality that only some people have. Resilience, on the other hand, encompasses attitudes, behaviors, and actions that everyone can acquire and refine. Research has demonstrated that resilience is commonplace rather than exceptional, and one explanation for this is the capacity to develop resilience. One illustration is how many Americans responded to the terrorist events on September 11, 2001, and how some people attempted to go on after such a terrible event.

Developing your resilience requires time and deliberate effort, much like developing muscle. By concentrating on four essential elements—connection, well-being, healthy thinking, and

215

meaning—you may strengthen your ability to endure trying times and painful events while also learning from them. Use these techniques to strengthen your ability to weather challenges and learn from them.

Develop your network

Place connections first. When facing challenges, connecting with sympathetic and understanding people can serve as a reminder that you're not alone. Find someone who will listen to you with compassion and trust, since this will help you develop your resilience talent.

Some people may want to withdraw themselves as a result of the agony of traumatic experiences, but it's crucial to accept support and assistance from others who care about you. Try to give priority to actually connecting with people who care about you, whether you schedule a lunchtime outing with a buddy or a weekly date night with your spouse. Assemble a group. Along with one-on-one interactions, some people discover that participating in community activities such as civic associations, religious communities, or other regional organizations offers social support and can help them regain hope. Look into local organizations that might provide you with support, a sense of direction, or joy when you need them.

Encourage wellness

Take good care of yourself. Although it may be a trendy buzzword, self-care is a valid practice for improving resilience and mental health. This is because stress affects both the body and the mind. Promoting healthy lifestyle habits like a balanced diet, enough sleep, water intake, and regular exercise will help your body become more resilient to stress and lessen the impact of negative emotions like anxiety or sadness.

Engage in mindfulness. Yoga, mindful writing, and other spiritual disciplines like prayer or meditation may also foster relationships and rekindle hope, which can better prepare people to handle adversity. Remember your blessings and express your gratitude even amid personal difficulties, whether you journal, meditate, or pray.

220

Skip the bad media. It may
be tempting to use alcohol,
drugs, or other substances
to dull your pain, but doing
so is like applying a bandage
to a serious wound. Instead
of attempting to completely
eradicate the sense of stress,
concentrate on providing
your body with the tools it
needs to manage stress.
Find a goal
Assist others. You may get a
sense of purpose, nurture
self-worth, connect with
others, and directly help

221

others by volunteering at a local homeless shelter or by just offering support to a friend in need. You can strengthen your resilience by doing all of these things. enhancing your greatest assets or updating your CV. Taking action can increase your probability of persevering through difficult circumstances again by serving as a reminder that you can find drive and purpose even in stressful situations.

Work toward your objectives. Create some reasonable objectives and maintain a consistent routine, even if it seems difficult. Take initiative. During difficult times, it's necessary to acknowledge and embrace your feelings, but it's also crucial to encourage self-discovery by asking yourself, "What can I do about a problem in my life?" Divide the problems into smaller, more manageable pieces if they seem too big to address all at once.

For example, if you're feeling overwhelmed by a difficulty, tell yourself that what occurred to you isn't a predictor of how your future will unfold and that you're not powerless. A highly stressful incident may not be something you can alter, but you can alter how you perceive it and react to it.

Accept change. Accept change as a normal part of

life. Negative circumstances in your life may make certain ambitions or ideals no longer reachable. Accepting the conditions that cannot be changed can make it simpler to focus on the ones that you can change.

Keep a positive mindset. It's challenging to maintain optimism when things aren't going your way. A positive mindset gives you the confidence to anticipate wonderful things in your life. Instead of focusing on what you fear, try picturing what you desire. Keep track of any slight changes in how you feel as you navigate challenging circumstances. Take lessons from your history. You could learn how to react skillfully to upcoming challenging situations by reflecting on who or what was supportive during earlier difficult times. Remember those times when you were able to rely on them and consider what you learned from them.

seeking assistance

Getting assistance when you need it is essential to developing resilience.

Building resilience may be as simple as using resources and the abovementioned methods for many people. On the road to resilience, a person may occasionally hit a roadblock or struggle to advance.

Emotional Intelligence

227

In the dynamic and interconnected world of today, intellect alone does not ensure leadership or life success. Emotional intelligence (EI) is a crucial, though sometimes disregarded, characteristic that distinguishes exceptional performers. This essential trait extends beyond the conventional intellect to include a person's capacity for motivating themselves, controlling their emotions, and mastering social skills. In this lively debate, we'll examine the importance of emotional intelligence, its components, and its profound effects on both personal and professional success.

Self-Regulation: Self-regulation, a key component of emotional maturity, sits at the heart of emotional intelligence. It alludes to the capacity to successfully restrain and manage one's feelings, inclinations, and actions. Self-control experts can remain calm and collected under pressure. They can make well-considered judgments even in trying situations since they are not easily persuaded by emotional upheaval. A leader with excellent self-regulation, for example, may handle a crisis with composure and poise, concentrating on solutions rather than giving in to fear. This skill not only builds team members' confidence but also a productive and secure work atmosphere.

Motivation: The inner force that pushes people toward their goals, motivation, is directly correlated with emotional intelligence. People with high EI are driven to succeed on their own and have a strong desire to do so. They foresee achievement, establish ambitious yet doable goals, and control their emotions to work steadfastly toward their goals.

Think of a competitor getting ready for a big match. During demanding training sessions, their emotional intelligence feeds their commitment and tenacity. Their success on the field is ultimately a result of their unrelenting motivation.

Another critical aspect of emotional intelligence is social skills. They cover a variety of skills, such as empathic reasoning, effective communication, and conflict resolution. People with high social skills can interpret social signs, modify their communication styles for various audiences, and form deep relationships with others.

For instance, a manager with excellent people skills may foster a supportive and cooperative workplace culture. They encourage a sense of camaraderie among

233

staff members by actively listening to their issues and providing helpful suggestions. This encourages a favorable working culture, which boosts morale and productivity.

Impact on Success, Both Personal and Professional: Success on both a personal and professional level is significantly influenced by emotional intelligence. High-EI people typically have higher stress management skills, are more adaptive, and are better at making decisions. They develop relationships with others on a deeper, more meaningful level, which enhances personal connections and increases their chances of career success.

Emotionally intelligent people excel as leaders in the workplace. They encourage a climate of empathy and understanding, support effective

235

communication, and inspire and motivate their colleagues. They are skilled at settling disputes, promoting a healthy work atmosphere, and encouraging innovation as leaders.

Additionally, emotional intelligence has a positive impact on both physical and mental health. Effective emotion and stress management helps people feel less anxious, more focused, and more fulfilled in both their personal and professional lives

Emotional Intelligence Development:

The good news is that emotional intelligence may be developed over time and is not a set trait. The following are some techniques to improve emotional intelligence:

Engage in mindfulness exercises to raise your level of awareness of your feelings and responses.

Gain emotional awareness by becoming aware of your emotional triggers and reactions in various contexts.

Ask for feedback: To learn more about how you come across in social situations, ask trusted people for their opinions.

Participate in activities that promote good collaboration and communication to develop social skills.

Set objectives: Specify specific, attainable

objectives and find the will to work toward them.

Practicing Mindfulness and Meditation

These techniques can help you unwind and lower your stress levels. Prepare your body and mind for sleep by including strategies such as progressive muscle relaxation or deep breathing exercises in your nighttime routine.

239

Limit caffeine and alcohol since they can interfere with sleep cycles and make the negative effects of stress on sleep worse. Try to stay away from these things, especially in the evening.

Make Your Sleep Space Comfortable: Make sure your bedroom is a relaxing place to sleep. Maintain a cool, calm environment in the room, and spend money on a cozy mattress and pillows.

Write Down Your anxieties: If you discover that your mind is racing as you lie in bed, think about keeping a notebook by your bedside to record your anxieties. By doing so, you may let things go and feel less anxious.

Limiting naps can help you get more rest at night, however longer or more frequent naps during the day might be detrimental.

Keep in mind that stress management and sleep

improvement are continual processes, and what works for one person may not necessarily work for another. Finding a mix of tactics that fit your requirements and way of life is crucial. If your attempts to improve your sleep are unsuccessful, think about consulting a healthcare provider or sleep expert for guidance. They can provide specific suggestions for stress management and enhancing your sleep quality in addition to assisting in the identification of any underlying sleep issues.

Managing Stress And Anxiety

Stress and anxiety management is a lifelong endeavor that involves self-awareness, perseverance, and patience. You may strengthen your emotional stability, develop emotional resilience, and handle life's obstacles with more ease and confidence by implementing these techniques into your daily routine. Living a happy and meaningful life requires putting your mental health and well-being first. The secret to effective stress and anxiety management is to discover what works best for you. Remember that everyone's journey is different.

Controlling anxiety and stress

Stress and worry have become frequent companions for many people amid the chaos of modern life. We frequently experience mental exhaustion and overwhelm as a result of juggling our work, relationships, income, and personal duties. However, we may learn to control stress and anxiety and promote a more balanced and meaningful existence by implementing effective solutions.

245

Knowledge of Stress and Anxiety

Stress and anxiety are physiological reactions that have developed to defend us against alleged dangers. The "fight or flight" reaction gets our bodies ready for danger, but in the modern world, it can be sparked by a variety of non-life-threatening circumstances. Understanding this instinct can help us spot when stress and anxiety are getting out of control and enable us to take preventative action to manage them.

Understanding the Symptoms: Early intervention requires an understanding of the signs and symptoms of stress and anxiety. Each person will experience these symptoms differently, but they might include irritation, restlessness, trouble focusing, muscular tension, headaches, racing thoughts,

247

and changes in sleep habits. We gain control over our mental health by being aware of these indicators.

Meditation and mindfulness

Stress and anxiety can be considerably reduced by engaging in mindfulness and meditation practices. Being present in the moment while accepting our thoughts and feelings without passing judgment is what mindfulness entails. Deep breathing exercises

248

and guided imagery are two meditation practices that can help relax the body and mind and increase feelings of inner peace.

Exercise regularly. Exercise has a significant influence on anxiety and stress management. Endorphins, the body's natural mood enhancers, are released during physical exercise and can reduce stress and improve mood. Exercises like walking, running, yoga, and dancing not only improve our physical health but also provide us with a way to let out our emotions. Adopting a healthy lifestyle is essential for controlling stress and anxiety. Our bodies obtain the nutrients they require to perform at their best when we eat a balanced diet that includes lots of fruits, vegetables, and whole grains. Equally crucial is getting enough sleep, which enables our brains to regenerate and absorb emotions efficiently.

Limiting your use of alcohol, caffeine, and unhealthy foods can also help you feel calmer and more emotionally stable.

Time management: Effective time management is essential for avoiding unmanageable levels of stress and worry. Prioritize your chores, set realistic deadlines, and divide your to-do list into manageable portions. To avoid burnout and maintain a healthy work-life balance, making time for leisure and self-care is equally crucial.

Setting Boundaries: A crucial strategy for controlling stress and anxiety is being aware of our boundaries. When you're feeling overwhelmed, practice saying no and aggressively communicating your requirements. Respecting your limits helps you feel in control of your life and lessens unneeded stress.

Getting Support: Getting help while coping with stress and anxiety is not a sign of weakness. To discuss your feelings and acquire insightful viewpoints, speak with friends, relatives, or a licensed professional counselor. Sometimes all it takes to feel lighter and relieved is to just share your ideas with someone.

253

Hobbies and Activities:
Taking part in hobbies and enjoyable activities can act as a pleasant diversion from pressure. Painting, gardening, reading, or playing an instrument, for example, all give you a sense of calm and achievement that might help you divert your attention from unfavorable thoughts.

Be gentle with yourself and stop talking negatively to yourself to prevent self-criticism. Keep in mind that tension and worry are normal aspects of being a person. It's normal to occasionally feel overwhelmed if you practice self-acceptance and compassion for yourself.

Chapter 6: Nurturing Relationships and Connection

Think of connections and relationships as fragile flowers in a huge, magical landscape. We must maintain our relationships and connections in the same way that a professional gardener tends to each plant for them to grow and blossom into something truly amazing.

Each flower in this enchanted garden stands for a distinct relationship we have in our life, from friends and family to coworkers and strangers. Just as every relationship is different and remarkable in its way, each one needs specific care and attention. We must sow the seeds of trust, empathy, and understanding if we are to cultivate these flower ties. We must talk freely and honestly with our loved ones regularly, much like we water the flowers, to make sure they feel heard and appreciated. We must share our joys with others, showering them with love and gratitude, just like sunshine does for the blooms.

Diversity is good for both the garden and our relationships. We may expand our garden by adding new plants (people), learning from their diverse viewpoints and life experiences, and therefore enhancing the overall setting. Accepting variety and being receptive to new relationships and friendships are crucial because they add to the garden's vitality and color. There are several seasons in this beautiful garden. Some relationships could go through challenging periods or disagreements, similar to how severe the winter can be. In these times, just as the gardener protects the flowers from frost, we must provide our assistance and compassion, fostering the healing of those ties.

Another virtue we get from taking care of this enchanted garden is patience. Similar to how not all relationships blossom to their full potential right away, not all flowers bloom at the same time. Strong and deep friendships require time and work to develop. Beautiful connections will inevitably develop with time and effort, so we must be patient and have faith in the process.

We and our loved ones change, just as the seasons do. The enchanted garden serves as a reminder to embrace relationship change and progress. People evolve, and with them, so do our relationships. We must be open to change, accept the changes that take place, and devise strategies for maintaining such ties.

261

In the end, the more love and care we put into these relationships and connections, the more beautiful and gratifying the landscape becomes in this enchanted garden. This enchanted place possesses the same healing, reviving, and great joy-bringing abilities as the secret garden in the old tales. We weave a magnificent tapestry of love and togetherness that will endure the test of time and leave a lasting legacy of delight in our lives through cultivating relationships and creating real connections.

Building Meaningful Connections

Creating meaningful relationships is essential for personal development, pleasure, and general well-being. It's a fundamental part of human interaction that improves our lives and gives us a sense of belonging. Whether it's personal relationships, friendships, or professional networks, meaningful connections bring us joy and fulfillment.

The key to forming deep friendships is authenticity. Being sincere and honest with yourself allows others to recognize and value the true you. Authenticity fosters trust and forms the foundation for deeper, more lasting connections. By being true to yourself, you can attract people who appreciate and respect you for who you are. So, always be yourself and embrace your unique qualities. It's the best way to form genuine connections that can enrich your life in countless ways.

It is important to actively listen when trying to create deep connections with others. When you listen intently to someone, it shows that you respect their views and feelings. This can lead to a stronger connection because it encourages empathy and understanding.

Empathy is the ability to understand how someone else is feeling and to see things from their perspective. By demonstrating empathy and support, you can build stronger relationships and establish trust. Another important factor in creating meaningful connections is sharing values and interests. When two people have things in common, such as beliefs or hobbies, it can help them bond and feel a sense of camaraderie. So, if you want to deepen your connections with others, try actively listening, showing empathy, and finding common ground.

I strongly believe that being honest and vulnerable with people is crucial to building deep relationships. It may not always be easy, but it is a powerful approach that communicates your emotional commitment to the connection and your confidence in the other person.

For a relationship to be strong, it needs honesty, vulnerability, effective communication, and mutual support.

Furthermore, support and encouragement are essential for developing meaningful partnerships. Being there for someone through both their successes and struggles demonstrates your sincere concern for their well-being and deepens the relationship.

Building Meaningful Connections Has Many Advantages

Increased Happiness: Positive relationships enrich our lives and make us happier people. Our general well-being is improved when we perceive people to be sympathetic, understanding, and caring.

Reduced Stress and Anxiety: Being aware that we have individuals to turn to in trying situations helps to lessen stress and anxiety. Meaningful relationships offer emotional support and can act as a safety net against the difficulties of life.

Better Mental Health: Making meaningful relationships can benefit mental health by minimizing emotions of loneliness and isolation.

Professional Success: In the workplace, meaningful connections promote networking, cooperation, and career advancement. Colleague and mentor connections that are solid can lead to new possibilities and help professional progress.

A more vital Social Support System: A robust social support system is produced through a network of meaningful relationships. The value of this network increases on happy and sad occasions.

Lifelong Friendships: Friendships that last a lifetime and frequently result from meaningful relationships These relationships offer companionship and a sense of community throughout all phases of life.

To summarize, making meaningful relationships requires us to be genuine, empathic, and helpful in our interactions with others. These relationships improve our lives and add to our general pleasure and well-being. Remember that genuine relationships take time and effort, but the benefits are priceless.

Healthy Communication

Healthy communication is an essential component of establishing and sustaining healthy and productive relationships, whether within a family, among friends, or in the workplace. It entails the courteous, straightforward, and productive sharing of views, ideas, sentiments, and information. Healthy communication is essential for dispute resolution, understanding one another, and cultivating a supportive and compassionate atmosphere. Here are some of the most essential parts of healthy communication:

Listening Actively: Being present, paying attention, and being interested in what people are saying while actively listening to them is essential. This entails giving the speaker your full attention and avoiding interruptions, such as checking your phone or planning your next move.

Respect and Empathy: Healthy communication entails treating people with respect, regardless of disagreements or points of view. Understanding and appreciating the emotions and experiences of others, even if you don't always

275

agree with them, is what empathy is all about.

When expressing your views or ideas, use "I" words to keep the dialogue from getting hostile. Say, "I feel hurt when..." rather than "You always make me think."

Be direct and clear: Avoid using confusing language or sending confused signals. Convey your views and feelings to avoid misunderstandings. Being forthright also aids in resolving conflicts quickly.

Maintain Calm and Manage Emotions: It is critical to maintain calm even during difficult interactions. Before answering, take a minute to breathe and collect your thoughts, especially in highly heated circumstances.

Avoid Blame and Criticism: Rather than blaming or criticizing others, concentrate on the specific behavior or circumstance that is creating concern. This makes it simpler to develop answers without putting everyone on the defensive.

Positive reinforcement should be used. Recognize and value positive actions and efforts. Positive reinforcement may encourage people to keep talking successfully and create a supportive environment.

Encourage candid input from others and be able to

take constructive criticism with compassion. Accept possibilities for personal development and progress.

Compromise and Flexibility: In many cases, finding a middle ground and being flexible in your communication may lead to greater results. Be open to changing your perspective and developing solutions that fulfill the demands of everyone.

Use Appropriate Humor: Humor can be a strong tool

for communicating, reducing tensions, and creating a welcoming environment. However, be sure your comedy is appropriate and does not denigrate or upset others.

Understand When to Take a Break: If a debate becomes too hot or emotions are running high, it's fine to take a pause and return to the topic when everyone is calmer and more composed.

Healthy communication is a skill that can be learned and improved over time. Individuals may strengthen their relationships and create a more pleasant and understanding atmosphere in their personal and professional lives by practicing active listening, empathy, and respectful expression.

Chapter 7: Creating a Healthy Environment

A healthy atmosphere is essential for general well-being and enjoying true health. It includes not only the physical environment but also psychological, social, and emotional components. Individuals may grow and reach their greatest potential by creating a good and supportive atmosphere. Here are some important factors to consider while attempting to establish a healthy environment:

Pure Air and Water: Access to clean air and water is critical to healthy health. This includes effective waste management, pollution reduction, and the implementation of sustainable methods to maintain natural resources.

Food that is both safe and nourishing: A healthy diet is vital for good health.

283

Encourage the availability and consumption of fresh, nutritious, and locally sourced foods to boost physical well-being and immune system strength.

Physical Exercise and Fitness: Creating conditions that encourage physical exercise helps motivate people to remain active. Access to parks, sports facilities, and pedestrian-friendly infrastructure promotes regular physical activity and minimizes sedentary behavior.

Support for Mental Health: Addressing mental health is equally important for enjoying true health. Creating a stigma-free atmosphere that encourages open dialogues about mental health and makes counseling and support services available can improve overall well-being. Human beings flourish in a supportive social context. Communities that promote inclusion, empathy, and healthy interactions can help to decrease stress and improve mental and emotional health.

Work-Life Balance: Organizations that promote work-life balance have happier and healthier workers. Flexible work arrangements, stress management programs, and establishing a healthy work culture can all have a substantial influence on an individual's overall health.

Access to Healthcare: Ensuring access to high-quality healthcare services is critical for optimal health. This involves both preventative measures such as regular check-ups and vaccines as well as early sickness treatment.

Nature and Green Spaces: Green areas and natural components incorporated into urban surroundings can have a soothing influence on mental well-being. Parks, gardens, and natural

287

landscapes may be places of leisure and regeneration.

Educational Opportunities: Having access to education allows people to make educated health decisions. Health literacy promotion can lead to healthier lifestyle choices and an increased understanding of health concerns.

Environmental Toxin Reduction: Efforts to reduce exposure to hazardous chemicals and pollutants can have a substantial influence on public health. This involves controlling industrial emissions, encouraging environmentally friendly goods, and decreasing the use of hazardous chemicals.

Practices for Sustainability: Adopting sustainable practices in all parts of life, such as energy saving, trash reduction, and environmentally friendly transportation, improves not just the environment but also personal well-being. Preparedness for natural disasters and crises can help lessen the impact on health. It is critical for resilience to develop comprehensive disaster response strategies and community support mechanisms.

Creating a healthy ecosystem is a complicated task that necessitates the cooperation of people, communities, governments, and organizations. We can develop a caring environment that promotes true health and allows individuals to live full lives by addressing many components of the environment, from physical surroundings to social dynamics. Finally, a healthy environment serves as the foundation for individuals to enjoy holistic well-being and prosper in all aspects of life.

Detoxifying Your Living Spaces

Detoxifying your living space is a method that entails making your surroundings healthier by eliminating or minimizing hazardous chemicals and contaminants. You can improve indoor air quality, promote improved physical health, and boost overall well-being by doing so. When detoxing your living environment, keep the following points in mind:

Air Quality in the Home: Indoor air pollution may be dangerous to one's health since it contains more toxins than outside air. Consider taking the following actions to enhance the quality of the air:

Ventilation: Ensure appropriate ventilation in your home to allow fresh air to flow. To eliminate smells and humidity, use exhaust

293

fans in the kitchen and bathroom.

Air purifiers: Purchase a high-quality air purifier to assist in the removal of airborne particles such as dust, allergies, mold spores, and volatile organic compounds (VOCs).

Plants: Use indoor plants as natural air filters since they absorb toxins and release oxygen.

VOCs are compounds that are released by numerous household items and materials, such as paint, cleaning agents, furniture, and carpets. Prolonged exposure to VOCs might result in health problems.

To reduce VOC exposure: Select low-VOC products: Choose low-VOC or VOC-free paints, adhesives, and cleaning solutions.

Test out new items: Allow new furniture or carpets to off-gas in a well-ventilated room before bringing them into your house.

Consider utilizing natural cleaning solutions such as vinegar, baking soda, or lemon juice instead of chemical-laden items.

Mold and moisture must be removed since they can cause respiratory difficulties and allergies. To avoid mold formation, follow these steps:

Repair any leaks: To avoid moisture buildup, address any water leaks in your house as soon as possible.

Maintain humidity levels: If required, use a dehumidifier to keep indoor humidity levels below 50%.

Cleaning Procedures: Traditional cleaning supplies frequently include hazardous substances. Choose safer alternatives.

Green cleaning supplies: Select environmentally friendly cleaning solutions or build your own using non-toxic materials.

Clothes made of microfiber: Cleaning with

microfiber towels is effective since they absorb dust and debris without the need for chemical cleansers.

EMFs (electrical Fields) should be reduced. Even though research on the health consequences of EMFs is equivocal, some people prefer to limit their exposure.

Limit the use of electronic devices. Turn off electrical gadgets while not in use, especially in bedrooms at night.

Maintain a safe distance. Keep your distance from technological gadgets such as Wi-Fi routers and cell phones.

Declutter and organize: A clutter-free environment not only promotes mental health but also lowers possible hazards. Select **Natural Materials:** Choose natural, non-toxic materials for furniture, decor, and fabrics, such as organic cotton, bamboo, or recycled wood.

299

If your tap water has pollutants or toxins, consider using a water filter to guarantee safer drinking water. dusty places for allergies and dust.

Remember that detoxing your living environment is a continuous process, and it's fine to start small. You can create a healthier and more inviting living environment for yourself and your family by making conscientious decisions about the goods you use and the air you breathe.

Sustainable Living Practices

Sustainable living practices are lifestyle choices and behaviors that strive to reduce our negative environmental effects while also increasing the well-being of both current and future generations. These behaviors include energy use, waste management, transportation, dietary choices, and other areas of everyday life. Individuals may help conserve natural resources, reduce greenhouse gas emissions, and maintain biodiversity by adopting sustainable living habits. Some significant areas of sustainable living activities are as follows:

Conserving Energy: Energy usage must be reduced to reduce greenhouse gas emissions and battle climate change. Sustainable living includes adopting energy-efficient equipment, shutting off lights and devices when not in use, and maximizing natural lighting and ventilation in the home.

Renewable Energy: Shifting away from fossil fuels and toward renewable energy sources like solar, wind, and hydropower is a critical component of living sustainably. Solar panels installed on rooftops and support for renewable energy initiatives can help

303

reduce dependency on nonrenewable resources.

Water conservation is important since it is a limited resource. Fixing leaks, using low-flow fixtures, collecting rainwater for irrigation, and being careful of water consumption in daily activities are all examples of sustainable living techniques.

Environmentally Friendly Transit: Using public transit, carpooling, bicycling, or walking instead of driving alone in a car can greatly reduce carbon emissions and air pollution. Transitioning to electric or hybrid vehicles can also help promote sustainable mobility.

Waste Reduction and Recycling: Minimizing waste output is critical to living a sustainable lifestyle. Recycling materials such as paper, plastic, glass, and metal, composting organic waste, and making

305

intentional decisions to decrease single-use goods are all part of this.

Sustainable Diet: Choosing a sustainable diet entails eating more plant-based foods, eating less meat (particularly beef and lamb, which have higher environmental implications), and supporting local and organic food suppliers. This helps to lessen the environmental impact of agriculture and animal rearing.

Conservation of Natural Resources: For a society to be sustainable, natural resources like forests, fisheries, and water bodies must be used responsibly and conserved. This involves engaging in conservation initiatives and promoting sustainable forestry practices.

Supporting Sustainable items and firms: Choosing environmentally friendly items and supporting firms with strong sustainability

307

practices may create positive market change.

Participating in local sustainability efforts, participating in community clean-ups, and supporting environmentally aware policies are all strategies to encourage sustainable living on a larger scale.

Education and Awareness: Raising awareness of sustainable living practices is essential for motivating people to make positive changes.

Individuals and communities can be empowered by education to adopt more sustainable lives and be more conscious of their environmental effects. Remember that making incremental, reasonable adjustments to daily life is more important than making big changes overnight. We can advance towards a more sustainable and ecologically friendly future if we all embrace these behaviors.

Minimizing Exposure to Toxins

Toxin exposure should be kept to a minimum to preserve health and well-being. Toxins are dangerous compounds present in a variety of surroundings, including air, water, food, home goods, and personal care products. Toxin exposure can cause a variety of health problems, ranging from minor irritations to serious chronic disorders.

Here are some helpful hints for reducing your exposure to toxins:

Dietary Guidelines: Consume a well-balanced, organic diet high in fruits, vegetables, and whole grains. Choose pesticide-free, additive-free, and preservative-free meals, as they can bring toxins into your body.

Filtered Water: Invest in a high-quality water filter to eliminate toxins from your drinking water, such as heavy metals, chlorine, and pesticides.

Avoid using plastic containers, particularly those containing BPA (bisphenol A), since they can leach dangerous chemicals into food and beverages. Choose glass, stainless steel, or BPA-free plastics instead.

Clean Air: Make sure your living rooms have adequate ventilation to reduce indoor air pollution. If required, use air filters, and avoid smoking or allowing others to smoke indoors.

Natural Cleaning Supplies: Choose non-toxic and natural cleaning products for your house. Many commercial cleaning products include dangerous compounds that can be breathed in or absorbed through the skin.

Personal Care Products: Read labels carefully and avoid personal care products containing parabens, phthalates,

313

triclosan, or formaldehyde. Choose natural or organic alternatives.

Lessen Pesticide Use: If you have a garden, consider using organic gardening practices to lessen your reliance on chemical pesticides and herbicides. Regular exercise and saunas can help your body detoxify by encouraging perspiration, which assists in the evacuation of toxins via the skin.

Limit Alcohol and Caffeine: Excessive alcohol and caffeine use can tax the liver, which is in charge of cleansing the body. Moderation is essential.

Cookware made of materials such as stainless steel, cast iron, or ceramic should be used since nonstick coatings can emit toxic vapors at high temperatures.

Antibiotics should be used sparingly, as they can change your gut microbiota

315

and raise the risk of antibiotic-resistant bacteria.

Reduce EMF Exposure: Limit your exposure to electromagnetic fields (EMFs) by using electronic devices sparingly and turning them off when not in use.

Test for Radon: If you reside in a region where radon gas is more prevalent, consider testing your house for radon and taking the required precautions to prevent exposure.

Properly Dispose of Hazardous Trash: To avoid environmental contamination, follow municipal requirements for the disposal of hazardous home trash such as batteries, paints, and chemicals.

Overall, being aware of the items and chemicals with which you come into contact and making deliberate decisions to limit your exposure to toxins may considerably contribute to a better and safer life. If you have specific health issues associated with toxin exposure, you must speak with a healthcare expert for tailored guidance and treatment.

Promoting a Positive Atmosphere

Promoting a pleasant environment is critical in a variety of situations, including the workplace, schools, communities, and even within families. A good environment promotes cooperation, creativity, and general well-being, resulting in more productivity and healthier relationships. Here are some fundamental ideas and practices for fostering and sustaining a happy environment:

Communication Clarity: Communication that is both effective and honest is critical. Promote candid dialogue, attentive listening, and helpful criticism. Ensure that everyone, regardless of position or function, feels heard and respected.

Set a good example for others, whether you're a boss, teacher, parent, or community leader. In your acts and words, demonstrate hope, compassion, and empathy.

Recognize and Appreciate: Recognize and celebrate the efforts and accomplishments of people and groups. Recognizing and expressing thanks for hard work may go a long way toward improving morale and motivation.

Build Trust: A positive environment is built on trust. Maintain consistency, uphold your commitments, and be dependable. Promote a culture in which individuals trust one another and feel comfortable discussing their views and concerns.

321

Encourage Collaboration: Create an environment that promotes teamwork. Encourage cross-functional or cross-departmental collaboration since it can lead to fresh ideas and solutions.

Provide Opportunities for Growth: Encourage personal and professional growth. Provide workers or members with training, mentorship programs, or chances to improve their skills and expertise.

Work-Life Balance: Recognize the significance of work-life balance. Encourage employees or members to take breaks and vacations and to emphasize their health.

Constructively Address Conflicts: Conflicts are unavoidable in every workplace, but how they are handled may make a huge difference. To guarantee that disagreements are resolved constructively, encourage open communication and teach conflict resolution skills.

Encourage Diversity and Inclusion: Embrace diversity and inclusion in all parts of your life. Create an atmosphere in which everyone is welcomed, respected, and appreciated for their diverse viewpoints and origins.

Milestones should be celebrated as a team or as a community, whether they be objectives, birthdays, or other major events.

Encourage Laughter: Laughter may help relieve tension and create a happy atmosphere. Encourage appropriate laughter and comedy, but make sure it is inclusive and not disrespectful.

Provide Assistance: Pay attention to people's well-being. Provide assistance and resources to people who are suffering personal issues or hardships.

Implement Flexibility: When feasible,

provide flexible work arrangements or timetables. This can improve work-life balance and job happiness.

Encourage a Positive Physical Environment: Make sure your physical area is clean, tidy, and pleasant. The environment may have a big influence on people's moods and productivity.

Mistakes are chances for development and learning, so learn from them. Encourage a culture in which mistakes are perceived as learning opportunities rather than sources of blame.

Remember that fostering a pleasant environment is a constant activity that needs the continual dedication and cooperation of all parties concerned. You can build a more peaceful, productive, and supportive community or workplace for everyone by cultivating a good atmosphere.

327

Chapter 8: Integrating Real Health into Your Daily Life

It's easy to become engrossed in the daily grind in today's fast-paced society, frequently ignoring our health in the process. However, putting our health first is crucial for living a happy and balanced life. Real health is a comprehensive concept that includes one's physical, mental, and emotional well-being and goes beyond simply going to the gym or adhering to fad diets. This manual will show you how to incorporate true health into your everyday activities so that you can prosper in every area of life. **Start Every Day with Awareness:** Each day should start with a little bit of awareness. Take a few minutes to breathe deeply, clear your thoughts, and establish positive objectives for the day ahead before

329

reaching for your phone or rushing into your daily responsibilities. Using mindfulness techniques can help you focus more clearly, feel more relaxed generally, and reduce stress.

Fuel Your Body with Whole Nutrients: Fueling your body with nutritious nutrients is a crucial part of actual wellness. Place a focus on eating a well-balanced diet that includes fruits, vegetables, whole grains, lean meats, and healthy fats. Avoid processed meals and excessive sugar since they can cause energy dips and have a long-term detrimental influence on your health.

Water is crucial for sustaining good health, so drink enough. Make it a routine to carry a reusable water bottle with you all day and to routinely drink water. Energy levels are increased, digestion is aided, and general physiological functions are supported by enough water.

Incorporate Physical Activity: Exercise is essential for both physical and mental wellness. Make a habit of finding an activity you like, whether it's swimming, dancing, yoga, jogging, or any other activity. Even a little stroll might be beneficial when done at lunchtime.

Prioritize Quality Sleep: Although it is sometimes underrated, getting enough sleep is essential for preserving true health. Create a relaxing bedtime ritual to tell your body that it's time to unwind, and aim for 7-9 hours of sleep every night. A good night's sleep boosts immunological health and improves emotional regulation and cognitive performance.

Effective Stress Management: Stress is a part of life, but how you deal with it may have a big impact on your general health. Include stress-relieving practices like deep breathing exercises, meditation, and time spent in nature. These techniques can aid in lowering stress and enhancing mental clarity.

Develop Healthy Relationships: Social interaction is essential for our well-being. Develop good relationships with your family, friends, and coworkers, and surround yourself with encouraging people. Emotional balance and happiness may be enhanced by having deep talks and spending time with loved ones.

Limit Screen Time: In the digital era, it's easy to spend too much time in front of a screen, which may be harmful to our health. Set limits and be careful of your screen use, especially before bed. Instead of letting technology take over your life, use it sensibly to improve it.

Gratitude is a potent instrument for actual wellness. Every day, take time to think about all the things you have to be thankful for. By shifting your attention from what you lack to what you do have, gratitude may help you feel happier and more upbeat.

Real health requires gradual and deliberate integration into daily life. Your physical, mental, and emotional well-being may be enhanced by implementing tiny adjustments and adopting a holistic strategy. Keep in mind that true health is a voyage of self-discovery and ongoing development rather than a quest for perfection. So get going now and see your life improve as a result of your perseverance and commitment. Live honestly to enjoy a more happy and healthy existence!

Setting Realistic Goals

337

A crucial component of both personal and professional development is the setting of reasonable objectives. Realistic objectives are within your reach, useful, and within your resources, timeframe, and capacity. Setting realistic objectives improves your chances of achievement, keeps you motivated, and prevents failure or disappointment. When developing realistic objectives, keep the following in mind:

Self-Assessment: Begin by identifying your advantages, disadvantages, and restrictions. Be truthful with yourself about what you can do given your present abilities, information, and resources.

Make sure that your objectives are clear and explicit. Goals that are too general are more difficult to pursue and track. Clearly state your goals and establish quantifiable performance standards.

Time-Bound: Give your objectives a realistic time range. This will assist you in maintaining your commitment and concentration while averting procrastination. Long-term objectives might be divided into smaller, more attainable milestones to make the process more feasible.

Study and Planning: Compile data and carry out an in-depth study on the objective you wish to attain. Recognize the actions necessary, the difficulties that might arise, and the tools you'll require. Your chances of success go up with a well-thought-out plan.

Recognize Any Constraints You May Have: Take into account any restrictions you may have, such as any money or time restraints, or any outside variables that could affect your objective. Verify that, given these constraints, your goals are realistic.

Flexibility is a must, but don't lose sight of the fact that things can change even when you set goals that seem reasonable. Whenever required, be prepared to modify your objectives, especially if unanticipated difficulties appear.

Set inspiring and motivating goals to help you stay motivated. It might not be the best match if a goal is either too simple or too difficult. Finding the ideal balance can help you stay committed to your goals and engaged.

Goal Decomposition: If a goal seems too big, divide it into smaller, more doable tasks. A sense of success and continued progress can come from taking things one step at a time.

Seek Assistance: Don't be afraid to ask friends, family, or mentors for guidance or assistance. Sharing your objectives with others may

343

motivate you and keep you responsible.

Track Your Progress: Keep tabs on how far you've come toward your objectives. This assists you in staying on course and making any required corrections as you go.

Having realistic expectations does not preclude you from pursuing ambitious goals, so keep that in mind. It involves striking a balance between pushing yourself and establishing realistic goals that further your achievement. Setting achievable goals will boost your confidence, keep you moving forward, and enhance the probability that you'll succeed in accomplishing your objectives.

Designing a Personalized Wellness Routine

Making a detailed plan specifically suited to a person's unique health and well-being requirements is part of designing a personalized wellness routine. It attempts to enhance general well-being, encourage healthy behaviors, and attend to any particular health objectives or concerns. The stages of developing a customized wellness regimen are as follows:

Consider Your Current Situation: Start by assessing your present way of life, health practices, and general well-being. Think about things like your level of physical fitness, diet, sleep habits, stress levels, mental health, and any medical disorders you may already have. This evaluation will help you pinpoint areas that require improvement and lay the groundwork for your wellness objectives.

Clarify your wellness goals by setting specific ones. Setting precise, measurable, attainable, relevant, and time-bound objectives will

347

help you stay motivated, whether your objective is weight loss, increased fitness, stress reduction, better sleep, or mental clarity.

Before beginning any wellness regimen, you must speak with your healthcare practitioner or another trained expert if you have any pre-existing medical ailments or concerns. Depending on the state of your health, they can offer tailored counseling and assistance.

Make a Balanced Diet Plan Nutrition is necessary for overall health. Create a balanced and healthy diet that is in line with your goals and takes into account your food preferences as well as any dietary limitations. Variety is critical to understanding fruits, vegetables, whole grains, lean meats, and healthy fats. Regular exercise Select an exercise regimen based on your fitness level and goals. Exercises for the heart, the muscles, the joints, and the flexibility of the body might be included. If you're new to fitness or haven't been active in a while, start slowly.

Make sleep and rest a priority. Good sleep is essential for healing and general wellness. Create a consistent sleep schedule and an evening routine that will be helpful. Before going to bed, take some time to unwind. Sleep for 7-9 hours every night.

Manage Stress Prolonged stress can have a detrimental effect on one's physical and emotional well-being. Include stress-relieving activities in your daily routine, such as deep breathing exercises, mindfulness training, or time spent in nature.

Addressing Mental Health Be mindful of your mental and emotional health. Engage in self-care practices

351

that relieve stress and help you unwind, such as writing, spending time with loved ones, engaging in hobbies, or, if necessary, seeking professional treatment.

Keep Hydrated: Keeping your body at its ideal level of hydration is crucial. Drink plenty of water throughout the day, and avoid sugary drinks and excessive coffee.

Track Progress and Make Adjustments: Keep a regular eye on your advancement toward your health objectives. If required, modify your regimen for lifestyle or new goal modifications.

Always remember that a customized health regimen should be adaptive to your changing demands and circumstances. Be gentle with yourself and celebrate each small victory you encounter along the way. It's also essential to ask for help from loved ones, close friends, or health experts if you struggle to stay motivated or require direction while on your path.

Overcoming Challenges and Maintaining Motivation

The ability to overcome obstacles and keep one's motivation high are vital traits that can help people achieve in a variety of spheres of life. Whether pursuing personal ambitions, professional efforts, or dealing with life's ups and downs, These traits could significantly affect a person's success and general happiness. The following is a discussion of ways to overcome obstacles and stay motivated:

Set Clearly Defined Goals: Set definable, attainable goals first. When you have a specific objective in mind, it is easier to remain motivated and dedicated to your goals.

If a challenge appears too big to handle, divide it up into smaller, more doable tasks. By doing so, you may approach each section methodically and feel successful as you finish each stage.

Remain optimistic: Overcoming obstacles requires keeping an optimistic outlook. Instead of getting caught up in setbacks, concentrate on the progress you are making. Adopt a growth attitude, in which setbacks are perceived as chances to develop and learn.

Create a Support System: Surround yourself with positive, encouraging individuals who can uplift you when circumstances are tough. A solid support network may significantly change how you approach and deal with obstacles.

Aim to be flexible and open-minded. Because life may be unpredictable, you may need to modify your plans. Be flexible and prepared to adapt your tactics as necessary.

Learn from Others: Draw motivation from those who have overcome comparable obstacles and achieved success. Learning from their experiences might provide you with insightful knowledge and keep you motivated.

Recognize and appreciate your accomplishments, regardless of how minor they may appear.

Celebrating these victories can increase your confidence and help you stay motivated.

Take some time each day to see yourself succeeding and overcoming obstacles to reach your objectives. This routine can support your motivation and help you stay focused on your goal.

Set Realistic Expectations: While it's important to have high dreams, it's also important to keep your expectations in

359

check so that you don't lose motivation by setting impossible targets. Gradual advancement can have an impact that rivals that of quick achievement.

Self-compassion exercises: Be nice to yourself and recognize that overcoming obstacles is a normal aspect of life. If things don't go as you had hoped, try not to be too harsh on yourself. You should have compassion and empathy for yourself, just as you would for a friend.

Continue to Learn and Develop: Look for opportunities to learn new things and get better at what you already do. Developing your skills and knowledge may boost your self-assurance and drive to succeed.

Stay persistent: Persistence is essential since it often takes time and effort to overcome obstacles. Remind yourself of your

361

objectives and the reasons you began, even when times are difficult.

Never forget that conquering obstacles and keeping motivation high require a journey rather than a single success. It calls for commitment, tenacity, and dedication to personal development. You may establish the mentality and behaviors required to meet obstacles head-on and maintain motivation throughout your trip by

362

adopting these tactics into your life.

Celebrating Your Progress

A crucial component of personal development and growth is acknowledging your accomplishments. It is necessary for retaining motivation and cultivating a good mentality to take the time to recognize and celebrate your accomplishments, whether

363

you are striving to reach personal objectives, professional milestones, or overcome obstacles. Here are some justifications for why acknowledging progress is crucial:

Maintains Motivation: Highlighting your accomplishments encourages you and serves as a constant reminder of the importance of your work. It supports your determination to continue on your quest, especially in the face of difficulties or disappointments.

Builds Confidence: Acknowledging your accomplishments, no matter how minor, helps you feel more confident. It strengthens your confidence that you can accomplish your objectives and motivates you to take on bigger difficulties.

Encourages Consistency: Achieving your final objective can be made less intimidating by celebrating tiny accomplishments along the way. It makes it simpler to maintain consistency and commitment by breaking down a difficult undertaking into small pieces.

Perspective-giving:
Recognizing success enables you to consider where you were starting from and how far you've come. It gives you perspective on your trip and enables you to see the work and development you've gone through.

Reduces Stress and Burnout: Burnout can result from relentlessly pushing yourself without appreciating your progress. You may unwind, recover, and reenergize by celebrating milestones, which lowers stress and enhances your general well-being.

Strengthens the Support Network: Sharing your successes and making progress known to loved ones and coworkers strengthens a network of support. It promotes praise from others and could even motivate people to work toward their objectives.

Promotes Gratitude: Highlighting accomplishments fosters gratitude for the chances, resources, and assistance you have been given along the way. Your entire perspective and sense of contentment with your path are improved by gratitude.

Remember that you don't need to have a lavish party to mark your accomplishments. Simple congratulations, gifts for yourself, or even just pausing to consider your accomplishments may be valuable. Here are some methods to acknowledge your accomplishments: **Reward Yourself:** Give yourself a treat you appreciate, such as your favorite dinner, a night out

369

to the movies, or a day off to unwind and rejuvenate.

Share Your Success: Let those who have helped you know about your accomplishments, whether they be family, friends, or coworkers. Their support and compliments might help your celebration even more.

Journaling: Keep a notebook where you may record your accomplishments, obstacles you've faced, and feelings

you've had along the way. This may be a fantastic method to recognize your successes and offer inspiration for the future.
Set precise goals for yourself along the way, and then mark each one off with a marker. These milestones may relate to time, particular accomplishments, or personal development.
Visual Reminders: To keep track of your progress, make visual representations

371

of it, such as a vision board or a progress sheet.

Do not forget that acknowledging progress does not include comparing oneself to others or determining success exclusively by the outcome. It's important to recognize the work you've done, the lessons you've learned, and the development you've gone through on your path. Celebrate your modest victories, embrace the process, and utilize your development as a springboard for even bigger achievements.

Conclusion

Recap of Real Health Principles

To sum up, real health concepts are crucial for living a happy and balanced life. We have discussed the essential elements of sustaining excellent physical, mental, and emotional well-being throughout our summary.

First, we stressed the need for a nutritious, vitamin-

374

and mineral-rich diet that is well-balanced. In addition to promoting longevity and supporting general physical functioning, a good diet also helps avoid certain chronic diseases.

Second, frequent exercise is essential for sustaining both physical and mental health. Exercise generates endorphins, which reduce stress and increase mental clarity in addition to increasing physical health.

We also underlined the significance of obtaining adequate good sleep. Restorative sleep helps the body to rejuvenate and is crucial for mental clarity, emotional stability, and general health.

We also talked about the need for stress management. Adopting stress-relieving practices like meditation, mindfulness, or hobbies may greatly enhance our well-being because long-term stress can have a detrimental influence on our health.

We also looked at the advantages of cultivating healthy relationships and making solid social ties. A sense of belonging and purpose may be facilitated through meaningful relationships and social support, both of which are essential for maintaining mental health.

The need for preventative healthcare, which includes routine checkups, immunizations, and screenings, was also discussed. Preventing or controlling possible health concerns can be greatly improved by early identification and management.

We may live healthier, happier, and more meaningful lives by embracing these actual health principles, which include a balanced diet, regular exercise, excellent sleep, stress management, social relationships, and preventative healthcare. We can lay a strong foundation for long-term health and wellness by prioritizing our well-being and making informed decisions. Always keep in mind that making little, beneficial adjustments to our daily routines may have a big impact on our general health and quality of life.

Embracing the Journey To Real Health

Accepting the Journey to Real Health is a life-altering choice that has a significant impact on our daily lives. Instead of focusing just on short-term objectives or quick fixes, holistic health takes into account one's physical, psychological, and emotional well-being.

We discover the importance of prioritizing self-care and the importance of providing our bodies with a healthy diet, consistent exercise, and enough sleep. We value mental and emotional health and look for methods to reduce stress, build good connections, and nurture a positive outlook.

The path to true health is not always simple since it calls for dedication, tenacity, and a readiness to change and grow

It's important to keep in mind that growth is not necessarily linear, even if we encounter challenges and setbacks along the way. No matter how modest, every advancement advances our development and general well-being.

Accepting the path to true health also entails getting rid of bad routines and behaviors that no longer benefit us. It entails making thoughtful decisions and paying attention to our behavior to make sure they support our beliefs and goals for our health. Furthermore, achieving true wellness does not require going it alone. Creating a network of allies and getting in touch with people who have similar goals may

383

inspire, motivate, and hold you accountable.

In the end, embracing the road to actual health is about the transformation that takes place along the way, not simply the final goal. It involves taking back control of our life, feeling more energized and alive, and discovering a deeper sense of contentment and pleasure.

As we embrace this path, we learn that true health is a condition of well-being that enables us to flourish and live our lives to the fullest rather than only the absence of disease. Let's start now, and with each passing day, we'll get closer to living a better, happier, and more energetic existence.

Acknowledgments

I am appreciative of your presence and willingness to study the complexities of well-being with me as we set out on this adventure to discover true health and everyday life. Our effort to comprehend the fundamentals of true health and how it affects our day-to-day lives helps us get to the heart of what it is to be human.

386

I appreciate the value of your time, focus, and commitment to finding a better and more fulfilling life via this inquiry. Your dedication to personal development and progress is admirable, and I sincerely hope that by working together, we may unearth insightful knowledge that will better both our lives and the lives of people around us.

Let's go on this journey with an open mind, empathy for

387

others as well as ourselves, and a common conviction in the transformative potential of knowledge and self-awareness. As we explore the regions of true health, may we discover the beauty of balance, the strength of resilience, and the wisdom of caring for both our bodies and minds.

I appreciate your participation in this journey. Everything depends on you being here.

Thank You For Reading
with grateful,

GABRIEL WILSON

About the Author

Gabriel Wilson is a well-known specialist in health and wellness who is most recognized for his breakthrough research on achieving true health via daily activities. Wilson has devoted his career to assisting people in achieving overall well-being through realistic and sustainable lifestyle decisions. Wilson has a love for inspiring others to live their best lives.

Wilson's book, "How to Experience Real Health: Everyday Living," presents a unique perspective on health that goes beyond diets and exercise regimens. He gives readers practical advice on how to develop better habits in their daily lives by drawing on his considerable understanding of diet, exercise, and mindfulness.

Wilson urges readers to have a positive outlook and a close connection with their bodies and thoughts by emphasizing balance and self-awareness. His ability to simplify complicated health issues into understandable and accessible thoughts makes his work appealing to people from all walks of life. Gabriel Wilson motivates readers to prioritize self-care, make wise health decisions, and realize their full potential for a full and rewarding life with his engaging style and relevant tales. For anybody looking to start a life-changing path towards enduring wellness, **"How to Experience Real Health: Everyday Living"** is a must-read.

9 798856 145259